Independent Lives?

Community Care and Disabled People

Also by Jenny Morris

ABLE LIVES: Women's Experience of Paralysis (*editor*)
ALONE TOGETHER: Voices of Single Mothers (*editor*)
PRIDE AGAINST PREJUDICE: Transforming Attitudes to Disability

Independent Lives?

Community Care and Disabled People

Jenny Morris

150th YEAR
M
MACMILLAN

First published 1993 by
THE MACMILLAN PRESS LTD
Houndmills, Basingstoke, Hampshire RG21 2XS
and London
Companies and representatives
throughout the world

ISBN 0-333-59372-3 hardcover
ISBN 0-333-59373-1 paperback

A catalogue record for this book is available
from the British Library.

Copy-edited and typeset by Povey-Edmondson
Okehampton and Rochdale, England

Printed in Hong Kong

Contents

Acknowledgements

I owe a great debt to those disabled people who agreed to talk about their lives. It means a great deal to me that they were willing to speak about such personal things and I hope that they feel I have done justice to their experiences.

I would also like to thank Nasa Begum and Bala Thakrar for carrying out some of the interviews with Asian people and to thank them and Millee Hill for talking to me generally about the experiences of black disabled people.

The British Council of Organisations of Disabled People were a valuable source of information and I would particularly like to thank their Independent Living Committee who spent a day with me exploring the issues with which the research was concerned.

Unfortunately, I cannot publicly name those social services departments and disability organisations which helped to put me in touch with potential interviewees as I need to preserve the anonymity of the interviewees but I gratefully acknowledge their time and effort.

The Advisory Group for the research project, Nasa Begum, Sally Baldwin, Etienne d'Aboville, Val Evans, Ann Kestenbaum, Jenny Owen, Jane Ritchie and Linda Ward, were truly supportive and I very much appreciate their expertise and experience. Nasa Begum, Frances Hasler, Mike Oliver, and Jane Ritchie gave me valuable comments on first drafts of the book.

Last, but by no means least, I am very grateful to the Joseph Rowntree Foundation for funding the research and for having faith in me as an individual researcher, unattached to any academic or research organisation.

JENNY MORRIS

Introduction

Community care is a major industry in Britain today. An important area of central and local government policy, it creates thousands of jobs for civil servants, local government officers, social and health professionals and other white-collar and manual workers. An army of academics and policy analysts have researched it, praised it, criticised it.

Definitions of community care, and the priorities given to it, have fluctuated over the years. Currently, community care can be taken to mean enabling people who fall into one of the four 'priority groups' – older people, younger disabled people, people with learning difficulties, and those who experience mental health problems – to remain living in their own homes or in small residential establishments which seek to be 'homely'. April 1993 saw the final stages of the implementation of the 1990 NHS and Community Care Act which made major changes to the financing and delivery of what is called 'care' and placed a greater role on local authority social services departments for coordinating services. Both health and social services authorities have been exhorted to incorporate 'user empowerment' into the way that they manage and deliver services.

This book is based on research which concerns the experience of one of the 'priority groups', namely adults with physical impairments below retirement age, but which raises questions and concerns relevant to all of the groups covered by community care policies. Amongst the many pieces of research on community care there is very little which takes the experiences of disabled or older people as the starting-point; there is even less which gives a voice to the experience of being in residential care, of being dependent on a partner or relatives for assistance, or the experience of using statutory services. It is this experience with which this book is concerned. The chapters in Part II are based on in-depth interviews carried out with fifty people, aged between 19 and 55, all of whom need at least some help with daily living tasks. An introduction to the Part gives more information about the nature of the sample.

Before examining these experiences, which are concerned with the reality of community care, we need to set them in their policy context. This is the aim of Chapter 1 which, in looking at the historical development of community care policies, and in particular their application to disabled people, identifies some of the key issues.

One of those key issues is the extent to which community care policies are compatible with the ideas of the independent living movement, a rapidly growing national and international movement amongst disabled people. These ideas, and their practical implications, are the subject of Chapter 2.

Chapter 3 completes the examination of the background to the experience of community care by examining the way that family members who assist older and disabled people have been constructed as 'informal carers' and the implications of this for both policy development and service delivery.

Having explored the experiences of the fifty interviewees in Chapters 4 to 8, Chapter 9 looks at the implications of the issues raised for community care policy and practice.

A political and ideological battle is being waged around the question of the assistance that some disabled people need in the tasks of daily living. This battle is being fought between government and national disability organisations, between social service authorities and local disability organisations, and, most importantly, within the daily lives of disabled individuals as they struggle to get the assistance they require.

The terrain of this battle is constructed by policy-makers and professionals and named 'community care'. But the initiative is being seized by disabled people and their organisations under the banner of 'independent living'. This book attempts to challenge the way that disabled people are treated within the development of community care policy and practice, demonstrating that the provision of the physical help that some people require to go about their daily lives is a fundamental human and civil rights issue.

A note on terminology

This book uses a social, rather than a medical, model of disability (see Chapter 2). Since there is common confusion about the terms *disability*, *disabled* and *impairment*, it is important to clarify what these words mean at the outset.

Impairment refers to the functional limitation(s) which affect a person's body, whereas *disability* refers to the loss or limitation of opportunities owing to social, physical and attitudinal barriers. Thus an inability to walk is an impairment, whereas an inability to enter a building because the entrance is up a flight of steps is a disability. An inability to speak is an impairment but an inability to communicate because appropriate technical aids are not made available is a disability. An inability to move one's body is an impairment but an inability to get out of bed because appropriate physical help is not available is a disability.

Disability therefore refers to the oppression which people with physical, sensory or intellectual impairments, or those who are mental health system survivors, experience as a result of prejudicial attitudes and discriminatory actions. People are disabled by society's reaction to impairment; this is why the term *disabled* people is used, rather than *people with disabilities*. The latter term really means people with impairments whereas the disability movement prefers to use the politically more powerful term, *disabled people*, in order to place the emphasis on how society oppresses people with a whole range of impairments.

The term *non-disabled people* is used rather than *able-bodied people* because the point is that people who do not experience physical, sensory or intellectual impairments are not disabled by the prejudice and discrimination which denies opportunities to people who do experience such impairments.

Part I
Community Care and Disabled People: Setting the Scene

1

Community care

This chapter aims to set the experiences which are explored in Part II of the book in the context of the development of government policies on community care. It looks in particular at the way that government policies in Britain have affected the services available to disabled people, placing these in a wider social context. The chapter begins to challenge some of the key assumptions underlying community care policy and practice, thereby also setting the scene for the account of the independent living movement in Chapter 2, and the analysis of the issue of informal carers in Chapter 3.

The origins of community care

Although the term 'community care' was first used in the report of the 1954–7 Royal Commission on Mental Illness and Mental Deficiency, the administrative potential had been laid down in 1913 by the Mental Deficiency Act which enabled both statutory and non-statutory bodies to make provision outside hospital for people defined as 'mentally retarded'. This potential was further encouraged by Section 28 of the National Health Service Act of 1946 which stated that, 'local authorities may, and to such extent as the Minister may direct shall, make arrangements for the care and after-care of illness and mental defectiveness'. Section 29 of the 1948 National Assistance Act then gave local authorities the power, but not the obligation, 'to make arangements for promoting the welfare of the blind, the deaf or dumb, or other persons who are perma-nently and substantially handicapped'.

The 1957 Report of the Royal Commission drew attention to what it considered to be outdated mental hospitals and to the stigma which attached to being a patient in one of these hospitals. However, its Chapter 10 – 'The Development of Community Care' – did little more than recommend the expansion of services under the existing permissive legislation. This was duly incorporated into the 1959 Mental Health Act but there was no mandatory obligation placed on local authorities to provide, or expand, such services.

Two important factors lay behind the more decisive action taken by Enoch Powell as Minister of Health in 1961, when he announced that the number of mental hospital beds would be halved by 1975, with most of those remaining being in units within general hospitals. From the mid-1950s new psychotropic drugs became available which created the potential for controlling behaviour through medication rather than incarceration. And throughout the 1950s it became more and more clear that the costs of the new National Health Service were increasing, with no sign of the let-up in demand for services which it had previously been envisaged would occur after the initial backlog of need had been dealt with.

A number of commentators expressed scepticism that anything other than a desire to reduce costs lay behind the proposed closure of long-stay hospitals. However, while this has remained a criticism of government policy on community care over the past 30 years, there has also been increasing concern about institutions and what they do to people, including some well-publicised public scandals of long-stay hospitals.

The development of community care policies has always been rife with conflicting viewpoints therefore, as is reflected in a key text on social policy issues published at the end of the 1970s. Kathleen Jones and her co-authors attempted to untangle the different meanings attached to community care as a policy objective, stating:

> To the politician, 'community care' is a useful piece of rhetoric; to the sociologist, it is a stick to beat institutional care with; to the civil servant, it is a cheap alternative to institutional care which can be passed to the local authorities for action – or inaction; to the visionary, it is a dream of the new society in which people really do care; to social services departments, it is a nightmare of heightened public expectations and inadequate resources to meet them (Jones, Brown and Bradshaw, 1983, p. 102).

While Jones *et al.* went on to state 'We are only just beginning to find out what it means to the old, the chronic sick and the handicapped', it is notable that this perspective was, and arguably remains, missing from the arena of political debate and policy development. Instead, the spotlight has been much more clearly focused on family members who provide support to elderly and disabled people. This has happened for two reasons, the first relating to the concerns of government, the second being the boom in research and pressure group activity during the 1980s around the issue of 'informal carers'. This second factor is discussed in some detail in Chapter 3.

Why have governments supported 'community care'?

Although community care policies were initially couched in terms of local authority services provided as an alternative to in-patient hospital care, the policy debate was soon dominated by the issue of how to encourage families to care for their members, particularly the increasing elderly population. By the 1970s it was quite clear that what policy-makers meant by community care was not so much care *in* the community as care *by* the community, to borrow Michael Bayley's useful phrase (Bayley, 1973).

From the earliest stages of the Poor Law through to the modern social security system, the state has always been concerned that any kind of welfare provision – whether it be given in the form of money or services – should not deter people from looking after themselves and their families. The expanding role for the Personal Social Services, which was such an important part of the development of community care, was clearly defined in these terms. As Richard Crossman, the Minister who introduced the 1970 Seebohm reforms, stated 'The primary objective of the Personal Social Services we can best describe as strengthening the capacity of the family to care for its members' (CSE State Group, 1979, pp. 103–4).

Some commentators on government policy during the 1970s identified the way that the state was keen to enforce family responsibility and the implications of this for service delivery. One academic wrote that 'even when family members cannot or will not provide care, the service is refused on the basis that they should do so. In practice then, some local authorities are still guided by the principle of family responsibility as enunciated in the Elizabethan poor law' (Moroney, 1976, p. 21).

And at the other end of the decade which saw the establishment of social services departments and the expansion of their role, Margaret Thatcher, speaking as Leader of the Opposition Tory Party in 1978, gave expression to the perceived importance of individual and family moral responsibility:

> We know the immense sacrifices which people will make for the care of their own near and dear – for elderly relatives, disabled children and so on and the immense pàrt which voluntary effort even outside the confines of the family has played in these fields. Once you give people the idea that all this can be done by the state, and that it is somehow second-best or even degrading to leave it to private people ... then you will begin to deprive human beings of one of the essential ingredients of humanity – personal moral responsibility (quoted in C. Hicks, 1978, p. 244).

Throughout the 1960s, 1970s and 1980s, community care has been the policy of successive governments, partly motivated by cost considerations, morally justified in terms of individual and family responsibilities, and given sociological support by research which showed the dehumanising effects of institutionalisation. The growing criticism of long-stay hospitals for 'mentally ill' and 'mentally handicapped' people was boosted by public enquiries which started with those at Ely, Farleigh and Whittingham between 1969 and 1972 and had reached twenty in number by the end of the 1970s.

During the 1970s, however, the scandals of institutional life were mirrored by the exposure of what was happening to ex-mental hospital patients, forced to live in sometimes appalling conditions in hostels, or on the streets. Every so often a story would surface in the media of a family being coerced to take home from hospital an elderly relative with whom they really felt they couldn't cope. Although these concerns did not find their expression in the kind of public enquiries which fuelled the attacks on institutions, they nevertheless had some effect. In 1976, the DHSS produced a consultative document, followed by the setting-up of a joint funding mechanism for community care involving health and social services authorities, and a policy document in 1977, which set out the intention that more resources would be available for community care services.

However, the International Monetary Fund crisis and the demise of the Labour Government in 1979 put a halt to any significant increase in resources, and the incoming Conservative Government's

White Paper, *Growing Older*, published in 1981, put the emphasis firmly on family, rather than state, responsibility for community care:

> The increasing needs of increasing numbers of older people simply cannot be met wholly – or even predominantly – by public authorities or public finance. This will be a task for the whole community, demanding the closest partnership between public and voluntary bodies, families and individuals ... Whatever level of public expenditure proves practicable, and however it is distributed, the primary sources of support and care are informal and voluntary. These spring from the personal ties of kinship, friendship and neighbourhood. They are irreplaceable. It is the role of public authorities to sustain and, where necessary, develop – but never to displace – such support and care. Care *in* the community must increasingly mean care *by* the community (DHSS, 1981, p. 3).

Nevertheless, although most people who needed some kind of support continued to receive that support from their family – as they always had done – the numbers in nursing and residential homes continued to increase. Partly this was due to simple demographic reasons in the form of the increase in the elderly population. However, there was also general agreement that, while government may have intended community care to increase and institutional care to diminish, in actual fact 'the community care policies of successive governments ... made little impact' (Hunter and Judge, 1988, p. 4). In spite of the government's declared intention of discouraging institutional care, there was a hundredfold increase in DSS expenditure on residential and nursing home care between 1979 and 1989 while expenditure on domiciliary services increased by less than three times.

The community care reforms of the 1990s

Throughout the 1980s pressure was building on the government to take a firm policy initiative on community care. There was increasing criticism of the fragmentation of services resulting from the organisational split between health and social services responsibilities (National Audit Office, 1987). Concerns were raised about the way organisational inefficiencies were preventing the most effective use of resources (Audit Commission, 1987). The increasing cost of residential care was highlighted (Working Group on Joint Planning, 1985) and a major review of residential care concluded that such provision should be only one of several options from which people could choose according to their particular circumstances (National Institute for Social Work, 1988).

The Audit Commission's report, *Making a Reality of Community Care*, published in 1986, concluded that although by 1984/5 £5.2 billion was being spent by the NHS, Personal Social Services and the social security system on the four 'priority' groups – 'the elderly, mentally handicapped, mentally ill and younger disabled' – service delivery was beset with problems similar to those identified by the Seebohm Report twenty years earlier – namely fragmented services, little innovation and poor service delivery. An additional problem was identified in the form of the 'perverse incentive' to residential care created by its public funding through the social security system. Increasing numbers of older people were entering residential care, not because they were making a positive choice to leave their own homes, but rather because the availability of social security funding for institutional but not community services, and the failure of social services authorities to make it possible for older people to remain in their own homes, created the incentive for profit-motivated entrepreneurs to expand the industry of residential care.

It was this increasing drain on the social security budget which really provided the government with the incentive to act on community care. As it pointed out on the first page of its 1989 White Paper, *Caring for People*, the cost of social security support for people in private residential care rose from £10 million in 1979 to over £1000 million in 1989. It was clear that there was no end in sight to this ever-increasing demand on the social security system and Sir Roy Griffiths, whose 1988 report was to form the basis of the 1989 White Paper and the current reforms, had been specifically charged with addressing this issue.

One of the reasons for the government's reluctance to act earlier on community care had been its antipathy towards increasing the role of local authorities. Nevertheless, the Griffiths Report concluded that local authority social services departments (SSDs) should take the lead on community care but that this role should be more of an enabler rather than a service provider. SSDs were exhorted to make maximum use of private and voluntary service providers. These ideas were adopted by the White Paper and implemented with the 1990 National Health Service and Community Care Act.

The concept of case management was employed by Griffiths, the White Paper and subsequent policy guidance (Department of Health, 1990) as a tool by which individual needs would be assessed by professionals and budgets deployed in the most cost-effective way. The 'perverse incentive' would be removed by the transfer of social security funds to local authority SSDs who would then have the responsibility of deciding whether an individual's needs could best be met by residential care or through the provision of community-based services.

The 1990 Act was implemented over a two-year period. The complaints procedures and inspection units which local authorities were charged to set up by April 1991, constituted the first phase, together with specific grants made available by central government for new social care developments agreed between health and social service authorities on mental illness initiatives, and for the support of voluntary organisations involved in drug and alcohol services (although this grant was then abolished in 1992). The second stage involved the development of Community Care Plans by local authorities, jointly with or in close cooperation with health authorities. These were first submitted to the Department of Health in April 1992. And finally, in April 1993, assessment procedures for users of services had to be in place, together with the separating-out of purchasing and providing functions within social services departments. Most importantly of all, the transfer of DSS funding of residential care was made to local authorities in April 1993.

Community care and disabled people

One third of disabled people are under the age of 60. For policy purposes this group has been separated out as one of what are now called the four 'priority groups'. To some extent this has happened because the other two-thirds of disabled people – those over the age of 60 – have always been included within 'the elderly'. During the 1960s and 1970s important progress was made in focusing on the existence and the interests of those disabled people who were not elderly, although the disadvantage of this was that when disability started to be defined as a civil rights issue during the 1980s, older disabled people tended to be excluded.

The initial result of the identification of 'younger' disabled people as a particular group was an increase in the amount of residential provision. The NHS had taken over 54 000 beds for the 'chronically sick' in 1948, about 85 per cent of which were occupied by people over the age of 65 (Royal College of Physicians, 1986). The conditions which people endured in these wards and long-stay hospitals was often appalling and the public awareness about the 'war disabled' which followed the Second World War created a particular focus on the inappropriateness of consigning younger disabled people to such places. Leonard Cheshire led the trend amongst a small number of voluntary organisations of 'rescuing' younger disabled people and offering them better-quality residential care.

The 1948 National Assistance Act had laid down the provision of residential establishments run by local authorities and by 1986 fifty-four local authorities in England and Wales (just under half the total) had set up Homes catering specifically for younger disabled people (Leat, 1988, p. 206). However these were outnumbered by the Homes run by voluntary and private organisations (of which there were 198 in 1986) and Younger Disabled Units run by health authorities (seventy-two by 1986).

Younger Disabled Units were a result of evidence in the 1960s of the extent to which disabled people below the age of 60 were trapped in long-stay geriatric hospital wards. The government exhorted Regional Hospital Boards to make specialist provision for this group and backed this up in 1970 by making available £3 million to be spent over a four-year period on building specialist units.

Residential provision for younger disabled people therefore increased during the time that community care gained in popularity as public policy, although in spite of this increase in specialist provision, it was reported in the mid-1980s that 'less than half of those aged 16–64 are in places which are supposed to cater specifically for them: the remainder are in old people's homes, psychiatric and geriatric departments and ordinary hospital wards' (Royal College of Physicians, 1986, p. 30).

Wider social and economic inequalities are an important pre-condition for this exclusion of disabled people from society and their segregation within residential and hospital care. Although job opportunities increased for disabled people during the Second World War, when 'the labour shortage was solved by the recruitment of women and disabled people to work in essential services, hospitals, factories, offices and on farms' (Humphries and Gordon, 1992, p. 129), in general employers are not willing to adjust a working environment designed for non-disabled people. The exclusion of disabled people from the workforce, which is a feature of industrial societies, has created economic dependency and social inequality (see Finkelstein, 1980; Oliver, 1990; Barnes, 1991).

The post-war period has seen the development of strongly held ideas about the dependency and inadequacy of disabled people. The application of medical expertise to the experience of impairment had an important role to play in this ideological development, but so too did the rapid expansion of disability charities and the way that people are perceived within the charity ethic. Both developments undermined the position of disabled people as autonomous individuals and as citizens (Oliver, 1990, see also Hevey, 1992).

The treatment of disabled people as unequal, inadequate and in need of expert care did not go completely unchallenged, however. The most important challenge came from disabled people themselves, as discussed in Chapter 2, but there were also forces at work at the policy-making level which sought to promote their rights.

The Private Member's Bill which Alf Morris presented to Parliament in 1969, and which became the 1970 Chronically Sick and Disabled Persons Act, was fuelled by the Labour MP's personal experience of the social and economic effects of impairment (Morris and Butler, 1972). His father was disabled by the unemployment and poverty which accompanied impairment, his mother-in-law by the housing conditions which worsened her physical condition and imprisoned her within her own home.

The assumption behind Morris's Bill was that disabled people had the right to participate in society but required society to take certain action to make this possible. This echoed the approach of the 1944 Disabled Persons (Employment) Act which was based on the 1943 Tomlinson Report's principle that the majority of disabled people 'are potentially capable of working on their merits in ordinary or open employment as long as appropriate training and services are available to make this possible' (quoted by Pagel, 1988), and the 1944 Education Act which specified that disabled children should be educated in mainstream schools (Oliver and Barnes, 1991, p. 8). Although, as a Private Member's Bill, the legislation was limited in what it could require, the Chronically Sick and Disabled

Persons Act did attempt to ensure that local authorities would provide services, aids and adaptations to people in their homes, and to inform themselves about the disabled people within their community.

The shortcomings in the implementation of the Chronically Sick and Disabled Persons Act have been well-documented (Borsay, 1986; Barnes, 1991). Arguably, these shortcomings were not just a result of local authority lethargy but were also heavily influenced by the increasingly dominant view that disabled people are in need of 'care', a view which discourages a recognition of their status as citizens and of the action that has to be taken to protect such status.

The expansion of the Personal Social Services was accompanied by the development of professional assessment of the needs of disabled people. Any rights to services which might have been created by the Chronically Sick and Disabled Persons Act were quickly subordinated to the professional's role as expert assessor of need and gatekeeper of scarce resources. The result, as Colin Barnes concludes, was that 'Throughout the post-1945 period the expansion of health and social services for disabled people has been constructed upon the erroneous belief that disabled people are not competent to make basic decisions about their individual service needs' (Barnes, 1991, p. 124, see also Wood, 1991).

The continuing importance of the role of the medical profession in services available to disabled people also meant that the assessment of their needs was dominated by the medical model of disability (see Oliver, 1991). Instead of focusing on the way that social, economic and political institutions discriminate against disabled people, the way the built environment acts as a barrier to their inclusion in society and the prejudice that individuals exhibit towards those with an impairment, health and social services professionals have focused on medical conditions and physical inabilities. Above all, they have focused on the individual and his/her impairment rather than society and its discriminatory attitudes and practices.

These underlying assumptions have had a significant impact on the development of services aimed at people with a physical or sensory impairment. Rehabilitation services have been dominated by the treatment of functional inabilities rather than a tackling of social and physical barriers (Beardshaw, 1988; Brechin and Liddiard, 1985). Throughout the post-war period, resources went into hospital-based services rather than community-based services

(Harrison, 1987). Other research has pointed to the way that medical expertise retained its role in the functional assessment of physical abilities and was in fact expanded through the introduction of the Attendance Allowance in 1970 and the Mobility Allowance in 1975, as qualification for both benefits depended on a doctor's assessment (see Barnes, 1991, pp. 100–13).

The needs of those with physical or sensory impairments who were below retirement age were given very little attention in the development of community care policies; for example, only one of the twenty-eight Care in the Community demonstration projects launched by the government in 1983 was concerned with this group (see also Beardshaw, 1988). When the Living Options Project set out in 1986 to document examples of good practice in the field of housing and support services for disabled people, it concluded:

> There are few alternatives for severely disabled people between the extremes of living in institutional care facilities and living with informal carers at home ... Despite the emphasis on community care for the past decade, and considerable documentation of service needs, there has been little resulting benefit for younger people with severe physical disabilities (Fiedler, 1988, p. 11).

Progress by default

Only 31 per cent of disabled people of working age are in employment (OPCS 1988). The social security system is therefore of considerable importance in determining the quality of their lives but in fact the way the benefit system works merely increases dependency and penalises autonomy (Barnes, 1991, p. 122). Disabled people are forced to emphasise their inabilities in order to get benefits which are set at a level which do not meet either their mobility or their personal assistance needs.

There was, however, one development within the social security system which has been of major significance for both individual disabled people's ability to live independently and for future policy developments in community care. This was the setting-up of the Independent Living Fund in 1988. The ILF came into existence as a result of pressure from disability organisations on the government in the run-up to the 1988 changes to the Supplementary Benefit system (brought in by the 1986 Social Security Act). Under the new Income

Support system disabled people were no longer able to claim additional payments for domestic support and the government finally recognised that some disabled people would not be adequately compensated by the new disability premiums. At the same time, there was some recognition that the mainstream benefit system was not flexible enough to deal with the particular costs that some disabled people had, partly because costs varied according to individual requirements and partly because many people not in receipt of income support had just as much difficulty meeting these costs as those who were in receipt of income support.

The ILF was therefore set up with a budget of £5 million over a five-year period with the intention that it would provide regular monthly payments to a small number of disabled people who had personal assistance requirements. Numbers qualifying were expected to be in the hundreds rather than the thousands (based on those who had qualified for the domiciliary care allowance). The Fund's scope included people who were not receiving income support (as well as those who were) but whose incomes were insufficient to meet the costs of personal care and domestic assistance.

Applications to the ILF, and grants awarded, dramatically exceeded the government's expectations. In retrospect this is not surprising for the estimates of those qualifying were based on those qualifying for a benefit (the domestic needs allowance) which was poorly advertised and had a very low take-up rate. Moreover, ILF grants provided precisely what many people wanted – the ability to purchase the assistance required – and knowledge about the ILF was spread rapidly by the disability movement. Within the first year of its operation it was clear that the initial budget was grossly inadequate. By the time the ILF was closed down in late 1992, its annual budget had reached £97 million and over 18 000 people were receiving ILF awards.

The Independent Living Fund posed not just a financial problem for the government but also a political one. According to the Department of Health's Policy Guidance, issued in 1990, local authorities are prohibited under the 1948 National Assistance Act from making payments of money direct to disabled people to enable them to purchase the assistance they require. Yet this is precisely what the ILF was doing. While some SSDs had made either direct or indirect payments to disabled people (see Chapter 2), the government has continued to oppose such a practice – ostensibly on grounds of accountability but a more important concern is the cost implications. Such a concern was merely confirmed by the experience of the rapidly increasing budget of the ILF. We return to the issue of direct payments and their relationship to the community-care reforms in Chapter 9.

What will the community care reforms mean for disabled people?

Virginia Beardshaw concluded a bleak assessment of the services available to disabled people by saying, 'But social attitudes towards people with physical disabilities are changing. In a number of important ways disabled people are becoming more integrated into the community. Public access is improving, and the rhetoric – if not the reality – of disabled people engaging as ordinary citizens in all aspects of public life has wide currency' (Beardshaw, 1988, p. 45).

Community care policies both open up possibilities and act as a barrier to this optimistic prospect. Some of the possibilities are explored throughout this book and the nature of the barriers will become clear in the discussion of the experiences of disabled people who have personal assistance requirements. For the moment, however, we can identify two aspects of community care policies which constitute barriers to disabled people's full participation in society.

The first aspect relates to the way that a rights-based approach towards meeting people's needs for support has been undermined by the community care reforms. Whatever the failings of the previous system (and they were many) the funding of residential care was through a system based on rights laid down by legislation and statutorily binding regulations, including a right of appeal. The new community care regime envisages that those who need some form of assistance with the tasks of daily living will be assessed by a care manager who will then have responsibility for purchasing services to meet the assessed needs. While recognition is given to the rights of disabled people to have control over their own lives, the policy guidance illustrates quite clearly the way in which community care in practice may not actually enable this. In particular, the increasing role given to professional assessment and the government's continuing opposition to direct payments act as major barriers to autonomy and independence.

Second, the focus on informal carers – which lies at the heart of the community care reforms – acts as a major barrier to disabled people being considered as citizens in their own right. The words 'disabled people' rarely appear these days in policy documents and discussion without the words 'and their carers' tagged on behind. The meaning which is given to both the concept of 'caring' and of 'informal carers' is a crucial part of disabled people's experience of a lack of autonomy. Before exploring these issues, however, (which are the subject of Chapter 3) we need to look at how the growing politicisation of disabled people has given rise to a concept – independent living – which is compatible with some of the rhetoric of community care but in conflict with most of its practice.

2

Independent living

Policy developments around residential and community care have been much written about and analysed by non-disabled professionals, academics and politicians but within their accounts there is little room for the experience of disabled people. However, in recent years the growing consciousness and organisation amongst disabled people has resulted in their voice, their experiences beginning to be heard. This chapter looks at the development of a social movement – the independent living movement – which has its origins in the resistance to imprisonment within institutions and which is currently engaged in grappling with the reality of community care policies.

Origins of a movement

The independent-living movement in Britain has its roots in disabled people's attempts to leave residential care. Institutional life has always produced forms of resistance, as is clear from the songs which are part of the culture of long-stay hospitals (see *Values into Action Newsletter*, nos 68,69), resistance which has been fictionalised in William Horwood's novel, *Scallagrigg*. However, it was the benevolent paternalism of the voluntary-sector residential homes set up in the 1950s which provided the context for demands from residents that they have more control over their lives and the establishments in which they lived (Finkelstein, 1991, p. 20). The *Cheshire Smile*, a newsletter published by the Leonard Cheshire Foundation, contained, during the 1960s and 1970s, expressions of a wish amongst some residents for greater control over their lives. The

Le Court Home, run by the Leonard Cheshire Foundation, was a particular site of struggle led initially by Paul Hunt who later wrote of how the residents insisted that they wanted 'to extend the range of control over our lives ... to choose our own bedtimes, drink alcohol if we chose, freedom for the sexes to relate without interference, freedom to leave the building without having to notify the authorities, etc.' (quoted by Finkelstein, 1991, p. 20).

Initially, the management committee refused to countenance such things and Paul Hunt and others made contact with two researchers at the Tavistock Institute in an attempt to encourage research which would support the residents' wish for greater control over their lives. Unfortunately, the research which resulted – Miller and Gwynn's *A Life Apart* – is one of the clearest examples of prejudice against disabled people. Having visited a number of residential establishments, Miller and Gwynn concluded that if someone enters an institution because of physical impairment 'they are displaying that they have failed to occupy or retain any role, which according to society, confers social status on the individual' (Miller and Gwynne, 1972, p. 80). They highlighted the significance of this:

> To lack any actual or potential role that confers a positive social status in the wider society is tantamount to being socially dead. To be admitted to one of these institutions is to enter a kind of limbo in which one has been written off as a member of society but is not yet physically dead. In these terms the task society assigns – behaviourally though never verbally – to these institutions is to cater for the socially dead during the interval between social death and physical death (p. 80; for further criticism of this research see Hunt, 1981, and Morris, 1991, pp. 130–3).

Paul Hunt and others agreed that society's reaction to those in residential establishments was to treat them as if they were socially dead, but vehemently objected to Miller and Gwynne's assumption that this social death was an inevitable result of physical impairment. Inspired by the Fokus scheme in Sweden which provided housing and personal assistance support for disabled people, a few residents managed to leave Le Court and move into their own homes.

In other parts of the country, disabled people were similarly trying to leave residential care. Ken Davis and Maggie Hines, for example, left residential care to live independently in Derbyshire, setting up the 'Grove Road scheme' – where disabled people occupied ground-floor flats and help was provided by tenants who lived in the first-floor flats (Davis, 1981). This scheme became an inspiration for others trying to persuade housing associations, housing departments and social services authorities to put together housing with personal assistance, although in fact Ken and Maggie soon found that they wanted more independence and moved on into ordinary housing.

It was out of these kinds of struggle that the Union of the Physically Impaired Against Segregation was created in 1974. The fight against residential care and for the housing and personal assistance services necessary for independence was a key foundation of what has become an increasingly strong civil rights movement amongst disabled people. The UPIAS constitution stated:

> The Union aims to have all segregated facilities for physically impaired people replaced by arrangements for us to participate fully in society. These arrangements must include the necessary financial, medical, technical, educational and other help required from the State to enable us to gain the maximum possible independence in daily living activities, to achieve mobility, undertake productive work, and to live where and how we choose with full control over our lives (*Disability Challenge*, 1, 1981)

Throughout the 1970s, there was increasing contact and a building of networks amongst disabled people who were attempting in their individual lives to gain access to the housing and support services they needed. In 1974, the first impairment-specific organisation was founded which was run by disabled people themselves. The Spinal Injuries Association was to become an important part of various campaigns around independent living issues. Its members are people who, becoming disabled as adults and only surviving because of advances in the treatment of spinal cord injury since the Second World War, are often outraged to be suddenly confronted with the segregation and discrimination that faces all disabled people.

However, other impairment-specific organisations, most of which were formed in the 1950s and 1960s, continue to be run by non-disabled people although many disabled people are active within them trying to wrest control of the organisation away from those who act on their behalf (see, for example, *Muscle Power*, a magazine produced by people with neuro-muscular impairment). Generally, however, the growing numbers of politicised disabled people have put their energies into local and national organisations which aim to represent people with all types of impairment.

During the 1970s and 1980s – when there was a dramatic increase in the number of organisations controlled by disabled people – the resistance to segregation in residential care provided an important impetus for a growing consciousness amongst disabled people of their rights as human beings and as citizens. Individuals involved in the Union of the Physically Impaired against Segregation (UPIAS) and later the British council of Organisations of Disabled People (BCODP), local disability organisations and organisations such as the Spinal Injuries Association have frequently acted as advisors and advocates for other disabled people wishing to leave residential care (see, for example, *Disability Challenge*, 2). Some local organisations of disabled people were formed in the context of opposition to plans by social services or health authorities to build new residential establishments.

A very important initiative was the formation of Centres for Independent (or Integrated) Living (CIL) which, taking their inspiration from the American CILs, aimed to provide advice and support to disabled individuals who wanted to live independently. The first CIL, and the best-resourced, was that in Derbyshire. In the early discussions with the County Council, the CIL was described as 'a system of services created by and staffed by disabled people, which could provide "the magic of peer counselling and peer models" serving people of all ages, whether blind, deaf or mobility impaired' (quoted by Davis, 1988, p. 15).

The concept of independent living was starting to take shape as both an aspiration and a principle which organisations such as the Derbyshire CIL wanted to inform the delivery of services. 'Independent living is acquiring the skills and support necessary for severely impaired people to have freedom to live where and how we choose with full control over our lives' (Davis, 1988, p. 16). The formation of the British Council of Organisations of Disabled People in 1981 provided a national forum for bringing together ideas on independent living and how to achieve it. There was also an important international dimension to the debate, through the Disabled People's International (also founded in 1981) and, by the end of the 1980s, through the establishment of the European Network on Integrated Living.

Many of those individuals now engaged at a local and national level in pursuing the goals of independent living have a long history of experiencing segregation and discrimination. People like John Evans, Chair of British Council of Organisations of Disabled People (BCODP)'s Independent Living Committee in 1992, have first-hand experience of years spent in an institution, and of the struggle to gain access to suitable housing and funding for personal assistance to make it possible to live in the community (Hampshire CIL, 1986). It is out of this type of experience that the concept of independent living has been refined.

The philosophy of the independent living movement

During the 1980s and early 1990s, the term 'independent living' has sometimes been used by health or social services professionals to describe initiatives which they have developed in the context of community care policies. Focusing on professional assessments of functional ability and inability, these initiatives often bear little relationship to the principles and practice of the independent living movement. It is therefore important, in the context of the research and analysis with which this book is concerned, to set out clearly the philosophy and practice of the independent living movement.

The philosophy of the independent living movement is based on four assumptions:

- that all human life is of value;
- that anyone, whatever their impairment, is capable of exerting choices;
- that people who are disabled by society's reaction to physical, intellectual and sensory impairment and to emotional distress have the right to assert control over their lives;
- that disabled people have the right to participate fully in society.

The concept of independent living is a broad one, embracing as it does the full range of human and civil rights. This means the right to have personal relationships, to be a parent, the right to equal acess to education, training, employment and leisure activities and the right to participate in the life of the community. Although those who are most active in the independent living movement have been people with a physical or sensory impairment, commonly in their thirties and forties, the movement is clear that its aims and aspirations are as relevant to those with intellectual impairments, to older people(including those with conditions such as Alzheimer's disease), and to those who are survivors of the mental health system as they are to the stereotype of a fit, young male paraplegic (see Morris, 1992a).

BCODP's Independent Living Committee is also concerned to address the concerns of black and ethnic minority disabled people and to ensure that these interests are represented within its organisation and to respect their separate organisations. Independent living is an issue which is increasingly being addressed by groups such as the Asian People with Disabilities Alliance and the Black Disabled People's Group.

The independent living movement's belief that disabled people's lives have value is asserted against the message which is given by the system of segregated and institutionalised provision. As Maggie Hines wrote in 1983, after she managed to leave residential care, 'Institutions were places people like me died in. The longer I lived there the more I realised I was one of society's social outcasts thrown onto the ultimate human scrap heap' (*Disability Challenge*, 2, p. 6).

Although the demands of the independent living movement encompass the full range of action that would need to be taken to enable people with physical, intellectual and sensory impairments, and those who have been diagnosed as 'mentally ill', to participate fully in society, the issue of personal assistance has traditionally been a key focus. This is not surprising for an inability physically to do things for oneself has historically created and still currently creates the risk of segregation and institutionalisation.

The meaning of independence

In developing the philosophy of independent living, disabled people have had to redefine the meaning of the word 'independent' (see Oliver, 1991, p. 91). In Western industrial societies, this term has commonly been associated with the ability to do things for oneself, to be self-supporting, self-reliant. When physical impairment means that there are things that someone cannot do for themselves, daily living tasks with which they need help, the assumption is that this person is 'dependent'. And in Western culture to be dependent is to be subordinate, to be subject to the control of others. Much of the literature on community care refers to 'dependent people'; most rehabilitation services focus on the 'independence' which is to be gained by maximising physical mobility and physical ability to do daily living tasks. Those who cannot do things for themselves are assumed to be unable to control their lives.

In the context of the economic inequality which accompanies significant physical impairment in industrialised societies, the need for personal assistance has been translated into a need for 'care' in the sense of a need to be looked after. Once personal assistance is seen as 'care' then the 'carer', whether professional or a relative, becomes the person in charge, the person in control. The disabled person is seen as being dependent on the carer, and incapable even of taking charge of the personal assistance s/he requires (see Mason, 1992, p. 80).

The independent living movement challenges all this. Simon Brisenden pointed out that disabled people are victims of an:

> ideology of independence. It teaches us that unless we can do everything for ourselves we cannot take our place in society. We must be able to cook, wash, dress ourselves, make the bed, write, speak and so forth, before we can become proper people, before we are 'independent' (Brisenden, 1989, p. 9).

Brisenden goes on to say that the independent living movement uses the word 'independent':

> in a practical and commonsense way to mean simply being able to achieve our goals. The point is that independent people have control over their lives, not that they perform every task themselves. Independence is not linked to the physical or intellectual capacity to care for oneself without assistance; independence is created by having assistance when and how one requires it.

Control over the personal assistance that is required to go about daily life is crucial, therefore, to the concept of independent living. It is this control which enables the expression of individuality. Linda Laurie, speaking to a seminar on independent living in Hackney, London, in 1988 described the different approaches to life held by people in residential establishments and those who have control over personal assistance:

Those people we visited or spoke to whose life was spent with groups of other people they didn't choose to be with, in buildings rather than 'homes', where toilets don't have locks and the staff don't knock before entering your room, said: 'We go on outings to the shops, church, seaside. We have our lunch at 12.00 [noon]. We have to be in by 10.30 p. m. We have to tell a member of staff where we are going when we go out'.

The individuals describing their experience of an Independent Living Scheme and what it meant to them ... said things like, 'I eat what I like, cook how I like and when I like. I choose my own company. I choose my own carers.'

The difference is between the words 'we' and 'I'. Controlling your own care enables you to have an individuality and not just be part of the 'we' whose mealtimes, diet, bedtime, etc. are dictated to you because you're 'one of them', 'the disabled', 'the client', 'the patient'. I believe the taking away the sense of 'I' or self is the ultimate weapon of control.

From this assertion of individuality then flows the assertion of disabled people's human rights and their status as citizens. As Mike Oliver says, 'To be disabled in Great Britain is to be denied the fundamental rights of citizenship to such an extent that most disabled people are denied their basic human rights' (Oliver, 1993). Control over personal assistance is necessary if those who need help with physical tasks are to achieve both human and civil rights, in other words not only the right to have control over basic daily living tasks (such as when to get up, go to bed, go to the toilet, when and what to eat) but also the right to have personal relationships, to seek employment, to engage in leisure and political activities.

The practice of independent living

A number of initiatives have been taken by disabled people, together and as individuals, which have made possible an experience of independent living for some people and it is worthwhile focusing on some examples.

During the 1980s the Derbyshire Centre for Integrated Living (DCIL) worked with the statutory bodies in their area to develop services which would promote human and civil rights. Their identification of seven primary needs which disabled people have, influenced the development of public services provision as well as laying the framework for the service which DCIL itself offered.

These seven needs are: information; counselling; housing; aids; personal help; transport; access (Davis, 1988, p. 27).

These needs are seen as fundamental to enabling disabled people to participate in society on an equal basis. They reflect the way that DCIL, in common with other disability organisations, is concerned with the whole range of barriers to independent living. Greater Manchester Coalition's more recently formed Young Disabled People's Project, for example, seeks to encourage self-confidence amongst young disabled people (counteracting the lack of self-esteem which results from the experience of segregated education), gives advice about housing and personal assistance options, and also gives young people involved in the project the opportunity to learn to drive.

In the area of personal assistance, a number of important initiatives have been taken by disability organisations which promote disabled people's control over the help they need. The Spinal Injuries Association (SIA) set up in 1985 its own Personal Assistants Scheme which provides personal assistants to SIA members to cover both emergencies and temporary requirements that may be created, for example by going on holiday or on a business trip. The personal assistants are trained by users of the service which is provided free to members who cannot afford the full cost; otherwise users are asked to pay what they can afford.

Independent Living Alternatives is an organisation, run by disabled people, which recruits, administers and supports personal assistance schemes for about ten disabled people in North London. It is just one of a number of local disability organisations which provide help with finding the resources for and recruiting and employing personal assistants. Greenwich Association of Disabled People, for example, employs a Personal Assistance Advisor who supports individual disabled people in establishing personal assistance packages and gives ongoing advice and help. Hampshire Centre for Independent Living publishes a *Personal Assistance Users' Newsletter* which goes to disabled people throughout the county and acts as an important forum for the exchange of information and a sharing of experiences.

In different parts of the country, disabled individuals have exerted pressure on local authorities to provide them with the resources needed to ensure independence, delivered in a way which enables them to have control over their lives. Many people assert that the only way to do this is for them to be given the money so that they can employ their own personal assistants. This was the case for Jane Campbell and Ann Macfarlane who together persuaded their local authority, Kingston-upon-Thames, to make a budget available which would pay for the help they needed. This allows 'each of us to arrange our own system of obtaining personal support, employing the personal assistants directly and controlling their conditions of services. In this way we retain full control over our day-to-day living' (Macfarlane, 1990).

In a survey carried out in 1991 the Royal Association for Disability and Rehabilitation (RADAR) found that 23% of local authorities responding made 'direct payments' to disabled people who then employed their own helpers. The majority of these arrangements will have been made as a result of individuals putting a case to their social services department for control over personal assistance. In addition, a number of organisations, including the Spinal Injuries Association, act as a 'laundering mechanism' for money to be channelled through them to disabled individuals from local authorities. This is made necessary because direct payments of this kind are in fact prohibited by the 1948 National Assistance Act.

Disability organisations have kept up their pressure on local and central government to recognise the concept of independent living and to develop policies which would translate the underlying philosophy into practice. In the context of the community care reforms this has included intensive pressure on the issue of direct payments and the future of the Independent Living Fund. The disability movement however, has continued to put a lot of its energies into raising awareness and confidence amongst disabled people themselves, many of whose lives are dominated by dependency on informal carers or segregation within institutions or 'special' schools. BCODP's Independent Living Committee recently organised two events, in different parts of the country, aimed at reaching out to people who have personal assistance requirements and who do not have contact with the independent living movement. One participant at the first event wrote about how it was attended by people with a diverse range of experiences:

> the presently institutionalised, those living at their parents' home, the
> home-leavers, those supported in such endeavours by professionals or
> peers active in the movement, those having used Community Service

Volunteers or volunteer systems as personal assistants, and finally, those determined to avoid institutional incarceration (*Personal Assistance Users' Newsletter*, August 1992, p. 3).

Community care or independent living?

Human and civil rights cannot be achieved if disabled people are segregated and institutionalised within residential care. However, living outside institutional care does not automatically mean that a disabled person has control over the assistance that they require. Those disabled people involved in developing the concept and the practice of independent living assert that using friends or relatives as unpaid carers means that the disabled person is unlikely to be able to play an equal role in personal relationships or to participate fully in society. Brisenden wrote that enforced dependency on a relative or partner:

> is the most exploitative of all forms of so-called care delivered in our society today for it exploits both the carer and the person receiving care. It ruins relationships between people and results in thwarted life opportunities on both sides of the caring equation (Brisenden, 1989, p. 10).

There is also the question of whether local authority services, delivered to people in their own homes, enable people to have control over the assistance they require. As Beardshaw concludes from her review of the development of community care as it has affected disabled people:

> For the last couple of decades, the principal function of the health and support services has been to provide assistance for families, friends and neighbours of disabled people who provide unpaid informal support, rather than providing services directly for disabled people themselves (Beardshaw, 1988, p. 142).

Services only tend to be provided directly to disabled people themselves when they live alone and there is evidence that such services are not delivered in a way which enables people to have control over their daily living activities nor are they enabled to play a role in the wider society. These issues are further explored in Parts II and III of this book but we can see already that the emphasis on informal care, which is at the heart of community care policy, is in direct conflict with the principles of independent living.

In this chapter and the previous one we have started to identify the extent to which community care policies assume that professionals and others take responsibility for disabled people. The independent living movement, on the other hand, challenges this assumption, questioning whether impairment itself creates dependency or whether it is society's reaction to impairment which creates dependency. The movement also challenges the more deeply held assumption – rarely articulated – which is so often held by non-disabled people: namely that disabled people's lives are not worth living. Miller and Gwynne's research on residential care was heavily influenced by this assumption, but so too was the boom in research on informal care which was to have an important impact on policy-makers during the 1980s. In order to complete the scene-setting for Part II and the analysis which follows in Part III of this book, we now need to look in some detail at the issue of informal care and how this relates to the concept of independent living.

3

Independent living and the debate on informal care

Over the past ten to fifteen years, 'informal carers' – that is, people who provide unpaid assistance to members of their family, or to friends or neighbours, who are elderly and/or experience physical, sensory or intellectual impairment – have been identified both as a social group and as a public issue. Community care policies have never been simply about making services available to people in their own homes as an alternative to institutional care; unpaid assistance given by family and friends has always been seen as a major source of providing help. However, this contribution has increased in both practical and policy significance in recent years and the key importance which the Griffiths Report, the White Paper *Caring for People* and subsequent policy guidance all attach to informal carers came at the end of a decade during which considerable public and professional attention was paid to the issue.

This attention was partly motivated by an increasing recognition of important demographic changes and the rapidly expanding cost of residential care for elderly people. We have already seen in Chapter 1 how the latter was a key motivation of the 1990 NHS and Community Care Act. The total public expenditure on both hospital and all forms of residential care for older people amounted to £5504 million in 1990 (McGlone, 1992, p. 26) and the prospect of increasing demands made on public services by this social group was, and is, viewed with a considerable amount of concern by government and civil servants alike.

This increase is also fuelled by demographic trends, in particular, the increasing number and proportion of the population which is over the age of 75. In 1951, there were 1.7 million people over the age of 75 (3.5 per cent of the population). By 1981 there were 3 million over-75 year olds (5.7 per cent) and by the year 2001 it is estimated there will be 4.3 million (7.5 per cent of the population). The number of over-85 year olds is also increasing – from 218 000 in 1951 to half a million in 1981 and will rise to 1.1 million in the year 2001.

However, important though demographic and cost factors have been in influencing the public debate on community care, there were yet other factors which have had a significant impact on how the issue of informal carers was posed. The beginning of the 1980s saw two developments which influenced the way in which informal care would emerge as a concern for policy-makers. The first was the identification of informal care as a 'women's issue' by feminist academics. In 1979 Janet Finch and Dulcie Groves presented a paper to the Annual Conference of the Social Administration Association which, as Baldwin and Twigg put it, 'transformed the existing debate on community care'. Finch and Groves's paper cut through 'the euphemistic language of "community" and "family" to argue that community care was esentially about the care provided by women; and it discussed the effects of caring on women's life chances in terms of equality of opportunities with men' (Baldwin and Twigg, 1991, p. 118). There followed a decade of research and theorising about 'care' and 'caring', dominated by a feminist agenda of challenging the economic dependence of women, which did much to highlight both the existence of informal carers and the nature of their lives.

The second development was the foundation of the Association of Carers in 1981. Although there had been a carers' pressure group since 1965, the particular way in which the Association of Carers (now called the Carers' National Association) represented both themselves and those that they cared for, made an important contribution to how the public debate on community care developed during the 1980s. The organisation played a significant part in the way that carers became more clearly identified as both a national pressure group and, at a local level, as a group to be consulted when policies are developed and implemented.

This chapter looks first at the public representation of informal care and carers, focusing on the implications of this representation for those who are 'cared for'. We then look in some detail at the research on informal care and the policy recommendations which have come out of this research, identifying the implications for the type of independent living issues which were discussed in the previous chapter.

Informal carers as a pressure group

The emergence of informal carers as a pressure group is perhaps rather surprising in that most of the research on the way that people look after their elderly parents, disabled spouse or disabled child recognises that those whom academics and professionals identify as 'carers' rarely see themselves as such. Instead, the tasks in which people are engaged – whether they are just 'keeping an eye' on someone who is forgetful or whether they involve physical help with the most intimate tasks of daily living – are seen primarily in terms of family relationships and the complex mixture of love and duty which they involve.

Twigg *et al.*, in reviewing the research on carers and services, wrote:

> The point is frequently made that many carers do not recognise themselves as such; the term is unfamiliar to them and, some would argue, at odds with how they perceive their actions, which they would regard as an extension of family or personal relations rather than in terms of being a carer, with its formal, quasi-employment overtones (Twigg *et al.*, 1990, p. 3).

The social meaning of the term 'carer' is not simple. Those who are identified as informal carers are primarily in this position because of a relationship based on kinship, marriage or friendship, and associated with love, with caring about a person. Yet their identity as carers is also based on the tasks which they perform and which when they are carried out by a paid worker in an institution or in someone's home also define the *worker* as a carer. The way in which carers – paid or unpaid – are defined by those who plan and deliver services has had an important influence on the way that informal carers have been identified as a social group.

The first pressure group which represented those who are now called 'informal carers' was the National Council for the Single Woman and her Dependants (NCSWD). Formed in the 1965, it grew out of the way that economic dependence by an adult on a single woman's earning capacity brought with it a high risk of poverty and was concerned with campaigning for the social security system to take account of this, a campaign which resulted in the introduction of the Invalid Care Allowance (ICA) in 1975. The ICA was intended to compensate for loss of earnings incurred when someone had to give up work in order to look after a relative. The terms of its introduction were very much the same as those of the social security provisions originating in the Beveridge Report, namely that married women were economically dependent on their husbands and did not need separate provision within the national assistance 'safety net' (Wilson, 1977). The ICA therefore was only payable to men and to single women and was not extended to married and cohabiting women until 1986 after a married woman carer, Jacqueline Drake, took her case to the European Court.

The eligibility criteria for ICA created a clear injustice suffered by married women, who in fact make up the largest group of informal carers. In 1982 the NCSWD changed its name to the National Council for Carers and their Elderly Dependants, in recognition of the fact that, as single women decreased as a percentage of the population and as the elderly population increased, looking after an elderly parent was becoming a more and more common experience for married women.

It was in the campaign for the extension of the ICA to married women that more attention began to be paid to the kind of situation that was created when an elderly parent needed personal assistance. Articles in newspapers, magazines, television programmes – as well as academic research, as we shall see – started to highlight not the *economic* dependence of the person being cared for but the need for tasks to be performed for them and the consequent restrictions on the lives of the person doing the caring.

At the same time attention was drawn to the situation experienced by women who were providing assistance to a disabled husband. Judith Oliver was married to a leading member of the Spinal Injuries Association, one of the new wave of organisations run by disabled people. The SIA attempted both to represent the interests of people with spinal cord injuries and to provide a space, through a national newsletter and local groups, for experiences to be shared. It became clear to Judith Oliver that the wives and mothers of men with spinal cord injuries were being expected to provide a good deal, often the whole, of the support required following discharge from a spinal unit and in the years after injury. Rehabilitation for people with spinal cord injuries was dominated by the encouragement of maximum physical ability and there was little attention paid to relationships and feelings.

The SIA ran a Link Scheme, putting newly injured people and their families in touch with others who had been through similar experiences, and it was partly her experience of involvement in this scheme which prompted Judith Oliver to write a letter in the SIA Newsletter in 1979 highlighting the difficulties faced by wives of men with spinal cord injury. She invited responses to be sent to her, care of the SIA offices, and it was from this initiative that the Association of Carers was then formed in 1981.

Initially, the SIA was closely involved with the new organisation. Its Welfare Officer was on the Management Committee, provided advice about fundraising and spoke on behalf of the Association of Carers in a number of different contexts. However, while the SIA's position was that professionals should not assume that families *would* provide assistance to people with spinal cord injuries and that services and resources should therefore be directed to the disabled individual to enable him/her to carry on the activities of daily living, the Association of Carers increasingly took the provision of unpaid help by family members for granted and insisted that services and resources should be directed at the informal carer.

Those involved in founding the Association of Carers had been very much motivated by a recognition that some situations were oppressive for both the carer and disabled person, and they aimed to empower such carers to refuse to continue providing unpaid assistance. Alternative, paid, assistance for the disabled person concerned was obviously a necessary part of any such empowering of reluctant carers and although sometimes the Association found itself supporting institutional alternatives to community care, generally the emphasis was on insisting that local authorities provided disabled people with the help they needed. However, as the organisation grew, and particularly as it became accepted by government as the official voice of carers, a change in the key people involved was reflected in a shift in attitudes. The focus was much more on enabling carers to continue their role – and such a role is of course based on the existence of a 'dependent person'.

By the end of the 1980s, it was clear that the interests of the disability movement and the Carers' National Association (as it became in 1988) were, at a very fundamental level, in deep conflict with each other. At an individual level, the interests and needs of disabled people and those who provide them with unpaid assistance may sometimes overlap but, at the level of pressure group politics, the way in which informal carers were represented fundamentally undermined the human and civil rights of disabled and older people.

Two particular aspects of this representation can be identified. The first relates to the social construction of disabled and older people as 'dependent people' and the way the Association of Carers was not only influenced by widely held social attitudes but also reaffirmed them. The second aspect, which was an inevitable result of the first, concerns the extent to which informal carers have become the focus of policy planning and service delivery – a development which owes much to long-held government assumptions about, and policy aims for, community care but which has been reaffirmed by the public representation of informal carers.

The social construction of 'carers and their dependants'

By the time that the Association of Carers and the National Council for Carers and their Elderly Dependants merged to form the Carers National Association in 1988, the term 'dependent' had become very much accepted as a way of describing all groups of people who received assistance from family or friends. Economic dependence was no longer at the core of the meaning of the term; instead, the image which was conjured up by its use was one of physical and mental incapacity. This partly occurred because of the concomitant public recognition of the incidence of Alzheimer's disease. Many people who were identified as carers were looking after people who were experiencing significant mental deterioration and were unable to do things for themselves not just in the physical sense but also in the intellectual sense. However, those experiencing this condition were, and are still, a minority of people receiving help from a family member, friend or neighbour. Other factors have been important in the social construction of 'dependent people' – a term which has such significant implications for the civil and human rights of disabled and older people.

Foremost amongst these factors are the general social attitudes which are held about both old age and impairment and which inform the development of public policy. It has become a cliché, but it is no less valid for that, to say that society is generally organised with the needs of young, adult, non-disabled men in mind. A key part of the way that this assumption underlies the construction of housing and the built environment, the provision of education and the organisation of employment, is the notion of what is normal. Both old people and those with physical, sensory and intellectual impairments are measured against normality and found wanting (see Morris, 1991, for a more detailed discussion). This reaction to the supposed abnormal experiences of old age and impairment is largely based on what such experiences mean to non-disabled and younger people, the medical profession historically having a key part to play in the social construction of the meanings attached to these experiences.

Mike Oliver (1990) and others have identified the way in which the medical profession's treatment of impairment has created a very partial understanding of the experience, the way it has focused on physical, sensory or intellectual functions, distracted attention from the way that society's reaction to impairment disables people, and encouraged an assumption that cure, or death, is the best treatment. Peter Townsend has written about the way that dependency in old age is structured by social and economic factors. 'Retirement, poverty, institutionalisation and restriction of domestic and community roles are the experiences which help to explain the structural dependency of the elderly' he wrote. Townsend argued that it is society 'which creates the framework of institutions and rules within which the general problems of the elderly emerge or, indeed, are "manufactured"' (Townsend, 1986, p. 53). And Fennel *et al.* argue that, as with the social construction of disability, much of the knowledge about and attitudes towards older people have been 'medically inspired and orientated' (Fennel *et al.*, 1988, p. 39). Social services professionals and policy-makers have been signficantly influenced by this medical perspective to both impairment and old age, so that, for example:

> neither social work nor health visiting have built an independent knowl-
> edge base for work with [older people]. Both their training and their
> practice followed a medicalised approach to ageing which gave secondary
> consideration to economic and social issues (ibid, p. 40).

The medicalisation of old age and impairment, and the cultural identification of both conditions as abnormal, whose only alleviation is cure or death, encourages the focus on individual inabilities – whether physical, sensory or intellectual. The image of a drooling 'vegetable', or the cantankerous 'old lady', who make unreasonable demands on long-suffering relatives, is not far away.

Unfortunately, the way that carers, as a pressure group, have identified their needs has not only been framed by these assumptions but has also reaffirmed the medicalisation of old age and impairment. The Carers' National Association defines a carer as:

> anyone whose life is in some way restricted because of the need to take responsibility for the care of a person who is mentally ill, mentally handicapped, physically disabled or whose health is impaired by sickness or old age (Carers' National Association leaflet, 1992).

Rather than highlighting the contribution that insufficient income and inappropriate housing, unequal access to health care, prejudicial attitudes, make to the difficulties which too often accompany old age and impairment, carers' organisations – in focusing on the needs of carers dealing with the consequences of physical and/or intellectual impairment – have obscured the social and economic inequalities which lie at the heart of those difficulties. In particular, instead of identifying the way that an inadequate income and inadequate (or inappropriate) services create the need for unpaid assistance, the public representation of informal carers has tended to take the need for informal care for granted and addressed the interests of those who fulfil the role thereby created.

Informal carers as service providers

Significantly, such an approach is not even in the interests of informal carers. The focus on carers needing the resources – rather than resources going directly to those who need personal assistance – has suited government and service providers very well for this approach assumes that carers will continue to do a significant amount of unpaid work. 'Supporting the carers' is not just a cheap alternative to the proper resourcing of 'care in the community'; it is at the core of the government's community-care policy.

Sir Roy Griffiths, in his report, asserted that the first task of public services was to support carers and that service providers should start by 'identifying such actual and potential carers, consulting them about their needs and those of the people they are caring for'. The Department of Health's Social Services Inspectorate, in a publication offering guidance to social services departments on how to develop a policy on carers, pointed out that at 1987 prices, 'the value of [the unpaid work which carers do] saves the State between £15 and £24 billion per year' (Department of Health, 1991, p. 13).

Although a lot of effort has gone into the development of services aimed at carers in recent years, carers are not primarily *consumers* of services. Rather they are *providers* of a service which saves considerable public expenditure and the aim of policy is therefore to enable and encourage carers to carry on such unpaid work.

The implications of all this can be seen in, for example, the types of services which are advocated by the Department of Health. Policy guidance on implementing the 1990 legislation assumes that informal carers will carry on providing unpaid help and that assessment and service delivery must be aimed at supporting this role (Department of Health, 1990). In 1991, the Department of Health's Social Services Inspectorate published a 'guide for practitioners', offering advice on how to set up services which would help carers. The introduction to the guide referred to the 'potential scale of the catastrophe if carers were to refuse to continue bearing the burden of care' (Department of Health, 1991, p. 7). The perceived cost-effectiveness of such policies is further illustrated by the fact that, of the forty projects discussed as examples for supporting carers, twenty-six had an annual budget of below £20 000 (at 1987 prices) and twelve relied on unpaid volunteers.

Silencing the voice of disabled and older people

The identification of informal carers as a social group with specific interests, accompanied as it has been by the social construction of older and disabled people as 'dependent', has tended to limit the opportunities for the interests of older and disabled people to be heard. While there has been a growing crescendo of government and professional rhetoric in recent years on 'user-involvement' in the planning and development of services, in practice such involvement has tended to be dominated by carers as an interest group.

An example of this has been documented in the evaluation of the Birmingham Community Care Special Action Project (CCSAP), an innovative local project launched in the late 1980s which, along with a number of other projects, has influenced government and professional thinking on community care practice. The written policy statements which initiated and framed the development of the project contained no explicit statement that families and friends should provide the majority of care (as the Griffiths Report had) but the Project was in fact based on this assumption (Barnes and Wistow, 1991, p. iii). Consequently, 'a very high profile has been given to work with people who care for those disabled by age, physical difficulties, learning difficulties or mental health problems (ibid, p. iii).

When it came to consultation with 'user groups', 'a continuing programme of public consultations with people who care for a disabled or elderly relative or friend has been the most high profile activity initiated by CCSAP' (ibid, p. 10). There was no direct work with older people at all and the – minimal – consultation with people with a physical or sensory impairment was focused on a review of day services (which tended to be seen anyway as 'respite' for carers).

The evaluators found that when they interviewed key professionals involved in the Project, 'the carers' consultations were the only model of user involvement they talked about when discussing this aspect of CCSAP' (ibid, p. 35). This is not an unusual feature of community care initiatives; its latest manifestation is the inclusion of a carers' representative on the Department of Health's special task force set up in the autumn of 1992 to help local authorities to implement community care, and an initial refusal to include a representative of disabled or older people.

Such exclusion is a fairly inevitable consequence of both the perception of older and disabled people as 'dependent' (and therefore incapable) and the insistence of policy-makers, professionals and the Carers' National Association that informal carers are at the heart of community care. Such a silencing of the voices of disabled and older people can only be to the detriment of their human and civil rights.

It must be said, however, that many people involved in supporting older and disabled people do not themselves see their relatives or spouses as 'dependent' in the sense of being incapable. Many informal carers are keenly aware of the human and civil rights of those whom they look after – after all, for many of them, it is love which creates the caring situation in the first place. Many carers do not represent their loved ones in a way which denies them their humanity; the problem is that the concept of 'dependent people' is now so strong that any other kind of representation is very often silenced or reinterpreted.

One small example of this was an article written by Maureen Oswin about her experience of caring for her terminally ill sister. She wrote a moving account of the loving care which she gave her sister for five years, graphically illustrating the way that service providers failed to meet either her sister's needs or her own needs for support. The article concluded 'I wonder when a strong voice will be heard for that group of people who are disabled by terminal illness' (Oswin, 1992, p. 17.) The title for the article, given by the magazine rather than by Maureen Oswin, was *The Carer's Tale* – something which it transparently was not. Instead, it was a story of two women's experience of the farce of community care – Maureen Oswin may have written it but her sister's interests and experience were as integral to the story as were her own; indeed this was inevitable for it is clear that Maureen loved and respected her sister, and therefore did her utmost to protect her quality of life until the day she died. But over the years, the voice of the 'cared for' has been so squeezed out of the public arena that it was too easy to attach the label of 'The Carer's Tale' to the story.

Having firmly identified those to whom they provide support as 'dependent people' the Carers' National Association now heads a coalition of various organisations pressing the government to provide a proper income for carers. Such a demand is seen by the disability movement as being against the interests of older and disabled people – first because it confirms their dependence on people with whom they have personal relationships and second because it involves resources going to the carer rather than to the person who needs assistance. As the Disablement Income Group said, in reaction to the launch of the CNA's 'Caring Costs Campaign' in 1992, 'It is our view that since it is the disability that occasions the extra expenditure it is the disabled person who should receive the allowance direct' (Disablement Income Group, Press Release, 25 November 1992.)

The demand for a proper income for carers is part of a shift towards identifying family members who give assistance to older and disabled people as being engaged in an occupation. Such an occupation is based on the notion of disabled and older people being dependent, a burden on those whose sacrifice should be rewarded. The representation of informal carers by the Carers National Association has resulted in a social construction of 'carers and their dependents' which assumes that either carers represent the interests of older and disabled people or, where there may be a conflict of interests that those of carers should be paramount. Jill Pitkeathley, the Director of the Carers' National Association, argues against the idea that disabled and older people should receive a care allowance to enable them to pay for personal assistance. Instead, such an allowance, she says, should go direct to the family member identified as a carer otherwise there is 'no guarantee whatsoever that the carer would actually receive the income' (Pitkeathley, 1989, p. 146). This not only assumes that a family member has been identified as 'the carer' but it takes away the opportunity for the person needing assistance to choose who should provide that assistance.

The pressure group representation of carers has thus moved a long way from its origins, associated as they were with an organisation, the Spinal Injuries Association, which is now a leading player in the independent living movement.

Feminist research and informal care

Social science research has an important role in informing policy debate and challenging public attitudes. Unfortunately, a significant amount of the research which has informed the public debate on community care – feminist research on informal care – has both silenced the voice of those who need personal assistance and failed to challenge general social attitudes about old age and impairment.

Laying the foundations for feminist research on informal care

Research on, and theorising about, informal care has emphasised its significance for women as carers and the effect that this role has on their participation in the labour market. When feminist academics started to address this issue in the late 1970s and early 1980s, they initially drew on the statistical evidence of the extent to which women were caring for elderly and disabled people which had been published in two surveys by the Office of Population Censuses and Surveys, one on women's employment in 1968 (Hunt, 1968), the other on elderly people living at home in 1978 (Hunt, 1978). Hilary Land (1978) and Mary McIntosh (1979) had both started to articulate the impact of community care policies on women's role as carers within the family, but Janet Finch and Dulcie Groves's paper at the 1979 Social Administration Policy Conference clearly argued that such policies were incompatible with equal opportunities for women. The Equal Opportunities Commission backed up this conclusion by asserting that women's role of caring for older and disabled people was inhibiting their full participation in the labour force (Equal Opportunities Commission, 1982).

The increasing attention which started to be paid to the issue of informal carers came at the end of a decade during which a strong women's movement had highlighted the way the sexual division of child-care within the family disadvantaged women in the labour market, and the way that the social security system both assumed and reaffirmed women's economic dependence on men. The debate on informal care was initially informed by the feminist analysis of women's role as the primary carers of children. The discussions on child-care had taken children's dependency on adults for granted and the focus was on the way that the sexual division of child-care made women economically dependent on men, and what steps could be taken to change this state of affairs. When feminists turned their attention to the sexual division of caring for older and disabled people they similarly assumed the dependency of this group and focused on the way in which women were made dependent by their caring role, searching for ways in which their economic independence could be achieved.

However, in the course of identifying women's role as carers of older and disabled people, the terms 'care' and 'carers' have come to be used in a way which excludes child-care and women's role as carers of children (unless they are caring for disabled children) from the debate. This was neatly illustrated when a conference was held at Kent University in 1985 whose purpose was to 'bring together academics from the countries of Scandinavia and Britain who had for some time been studying and theorising on the concept of "care"' (Ungerson, 1990, p. 1.) As Clare Ungerson wrote:

there was some puzzlement on both sides of the linguistic and geographical divide as to why a conference on 'Cross-national perspectives on gender and community care' should bring together, on the part of the Scandinavian participants, both child-care analysts and commentators on the care of the dependent elderly, whereas, amongst the British participants, the term 'caring' had come to have a much narrower and more specific meaning, referring to the care of the incapacitated only (ibid, p. 179).

Undoubtedly, part of the explanation for these different interpretations was that the feminist debate in Britain addressed itself to a particular set of British government policies on community care which are concerned with older and disabled people, and not with issues of child-care. However, it is also significant that British feminist research and theorising on 'caring' was solely motivated by the assertion that community care policies were against the interests of 'women' (by which was meant non-elderly, non-disabled women). While the 1980s saw increasing attention in Britain on the rights of children it was not until the end of the 1980s that the disability movement started to make an impact on the academic consciousness in terms of the rights of disabled people. The failure to recognise the interests of older and disabled people meant that British feminist academics were able to discuss community care as an issue solely in terms of its effects on non-disabled, non-elderly women who were identified as shouldering a 'burden of care'. In contrast, Scandinavian countries have a longer history of recognising the civil rights of disabled people and in Sweden in particular, personal assistance services have been available since the 1930s (Ratzka, 1986). Kari Waerness's contribution to the 1985 Conference, entitled 'Informal and formal care in old age [in Scandinavia]' was notable for including a much clearer representation of the voice of older people than that contained in any of the British contributions.

Unspoken prejudices

From the early 1980s onwards, with the interests of non-disabled, non-elderly women firmly at the centre of the debate, British feminist academics who turned their attention to community care constructed older and disabled people as 'dependent people', focusing on the 'burden of care' which was imposed on women within the family. Before looking at the way that this research developed and its implications for the public debate on community care, we need to confront the assumptions which influenced both the theory and the research methodology.

We have already discussed the prejudicial social attitudes which are commonly held about older and disabled people. Feminist academics are no more immune from these prejudices than any other social group. At the core of attitudes towards older and disabled people is the feeling that their quality of life is often so poor that their lives are not worth living. This assumption is rarely articulated within the academic literature but it is nevertheless often there in the background. Dulcie Groves, who co-edited the key feminist text on informal care which is discussed below, wrote in 1979:

> If inadequate care is available to frail elderly people, some might prefer death as an alternative to cruel and pointless suffering. It seems a logical alternative ... In the absence of protective legislation for elderly and handicapped people, perhaps the least that can be done is to offer them a dignified way of ending what, after all, must be a living death (Groves, 1979).

Miller and Gwynne, in their research on residential care, categorised disabled people as 'socially dead', asserting that bringing about physical death was the logical course of action. Such a conclusion is only possible because of the assumption that impairment itself is the cause of such 'social death' rather than society's reaction to impairment. The same assumption often underlies research on informal care, namely that old age and impairment inevitably bring with them a poor quality of life and an inability to participate in society. Taking this for granted, attention is then focused on the difficulties experienced by family members who provide help and support to older and disabled people.

The construction of 'women' and 'dependent people'

When Janet Finch and Dulcie Groves edited *A Labour of Love*, a book published in 1983 which brought together the thinking at that time on the issue, it was subtitled *Women, Work and Caring*, illustrating the way that the key theoretical and political questions were focused on how caring restricted women's opportunities for paid employment. The dependency of those being cared for was taken for granted and the emphasis of the book was 'upon the tension between women's economic independence ... and their traditional role as front-line, unpaid "carers"'. The book was concerned with exploring the 'different facets of women's experience of caring, the dilemmas which caring poses for women, the tension between paid work and unpaid caring (which can be hard work) and the social policy issues raised by the particular topics under discussion' (Finch and Groves, 1983, p. 2). There was no room here for exploring either the experiences of older and disabled people or the social policy issues from their point of view.

A companion book to *A Labour of Love* was published, edited by Judith Oliver and Anna Briggs, both of whom were involved in the Association of Carers. While this book, *Caring: Experiences of looking after disabled relatives* contained powerful and moving accounts of the reality of 'community care' for those who had to care with little or no support from public services, it also clearly represented those who are cared for as 'dependents'. In asserting that informal carers were an oppressed group, ignored by policy-makers and service-deliverers, neither books left any room for the voices of those who were receiving care.

There followed a number of pieces of qualitative research (e.g. Ungerson, 1987; Lewis and Meredith, 1988; Hicks, 1988; Glendinning, 1992) which did much to explore and bring out into the open the experience of what it was like to be an informal carer. However, although this research purported to explore the 'caring relationship' not one study actually interviewed those who were cared for; instead such research was entirely confined to the subjective reality of informal carers.

The absence of the voice of older and disabled people from the research confirmed them as dependent people and undermined their humanity. This was reflected also in a number of articles and books which further developed a feminist analysis of caring and community care. Hilary Graham, in discussing what was meant by the term 'caring', emphasised that it involved not just 'feeling concern for' but also 'taking charge' of others (Graham, 1983, p. 13). What was not made explicit was that this 'taking charge of' element in the definition of caring is predicated on an unequal relationship between carer and cared-for (echoing the unequal relationship between service-providers and older and disabled people). The terms in which feminist academics wrote about older and disabled people, the way that they were given no voice and were constructed as dependent people, flowed naturally from both the shift away from looking at child-care issues to looking at issues around the care of adults, and from the general assumption that older and disabled people are 'other', not normal, not 'one of us'. Indeed, the language that was used clearly identified the interests of the feminist academic with the interests of the woman carer whilst there was no similar identification with the interests of older and disabled people (see Morris, 1991, pp. 154–6). In the process, not only were disabled and older people constructed as dependent people but the category, women, was constructed as non-disabled and non-elderly. There was no recognition that women make up the majority of disabled and older people, nor indeed that many disabled and older people are also informal carers.

Residential care as an equal opportunities solution

This failure to identify with the interests of older and disabled people was clearly illustrated when feminists came to articulate what they perceived to be the equal opportunities issues raised by community care policies. If women's caring role made them economically dependent, and community care policies were likely to confirm women's role as carers, should such policies be supported, they asked? As Janet Finch wrote in an article published in 1984, 'We are clear what we want to reject: we reject so-called community care policies which depend on the substantial and consistent input of women's unpaid labour in the home, whilst at the same time effectively excluding them from the labour market and reinforcing their economic and personal dependence upon men' (Finch, 1984). She then went on to ask 'Can we envisage any version of community care which is not sexist?' Finch has consistently argued that it is not possible to do so.

Feminist academics' identification of the equal opportunities issues raised by community care policies was entirely concerned with the interests of those women identified as informal carers. The attention paid to community care during the early-to-mid-1980s failed to consider whether there were equal opportunities issues for those who needed assistance (a majority of whom are women) and it is perhaps not surprising therefore that some feminists, such as Janet

Finch and Gillian Dalley, found themselves advocating residential care for older and disabled people (see Morris, 1991, pp. 152–3; 157–63, for a discussion of Gillian Dalley's work).

Janet Finch, in a paper published in 1990, argued that feminists should concern themselves with promoting what she called 'different models for the care of dependent people.' (Finch, 1990, p. 54) She acknowledged that one obvious response to the identification of the sexual division of caring within the family is to encourage men to take on more of the caring tasks, and recognised that this might be done partly through increasing the financial support to carers and partly through challenging the notion of caring being women's work. However, Finch is sceptical about whether this would ever be possible, and even if it were, she says, 'it might not necessarily be a state of affairs which feminists would want to support, partly because it keeps caring for dependent people in the family domain as a privatised activity, and partly because one would want to defend the right of women who need care to be cared for by other women, not by men' (Finch, 1990, p. 54). Significantly, this latter point is not based on any research about whether women who need assistance would rather receive that assistance in a family (where it may often be given by male partners) or a residential setting; in fact Querishi and Walker's research indicates that spouses/partners are the preferred carers of both men and women (Qureshi and Walker, 1989).

Finch goes on to argue that the feminist challenge is the assertion that 'community care need not mean family care' (Finch, 1990, p. 55). Although this statement seems similar to those made by activists within the independent living movement, what Finch actually means by this is 'new' forms of residential care. Thus:

> Policies devised on the basis of non-family care 'in' the community would have to concern themselves with how to provide a range of residential facilities, with nursing and domestic support attached, which would enable elderly and handicapped [*sic*] people to lead as independent and normal lives as possible, but in which the care would be provided by people who are properly paid for doing so. The de-emphasising of family care as the central feature of community care might well receive the support of handicapped people themselves, for whom personal independence is a key goal ... Of course within such settings attention would need to be paid to enabling people to maintain links with people (relatives or friends) to whom they are emotionally close, that is, people who care 'about' them; but in my view, removing the compulsion to perform the

labour of caring 'for' one's relatives is likely to facilitate rather than to obstruct that (Finch, 1990, p. 55).

While the construction of older and disabled people as dependent people developed partly out of the identification of child-care as an equal opportunities issue for women, the subsequent development of research and analysis on caring as solely concerning the care of older and disabled people is also reflected in the different policy implications which feminists such as Finch and Dalley have identified. Feminists have not advocated that the solution to the sexual division of child-care within the family is to confine children to residential care (unless they have a physical or intellectual impairment). Instead they have focused on the need to challenge men's attitudes to child-care, and have pressed for better nursery and after-school provision and for workplace practices to change to take account of the need for parents to look after their children. Undoubtedly, the generally prejudicial attitudes towards older and disabled people – which undermine their human and civil rights – had an important influence on the ability of feminists such as Finch and Dalley to feel that a denial of a home and family life were appropriate social reactions to growing older or experiencing physical, sensory or intellectual impairment.

An analytical straitjacket

Finch and Dalley – in their explicit espousal of residential care – do go further than many other feminist academics writing about community care. Other writers have tended to shy away from what is in fact merely the logical conclusion of the way their analysis is shaped solely by the economic interests of non-disabled women. Indeed in the past few years, feminist academics have started to acknowledge the interests of disabled people in response to the growing political voice of the disability movement (e.g. Baldwin and Twigg, 1991). However, the way in which the analytical framework for research on informal care has developed has acted as a straitjacket, as a limitation on how far feminists are able to go in recognising the interests of older and disabled people.

The construction of older and disabled people as dependent people means that they are treated as incapable. The focus therefore remains on informal carers and the only alternative to residential care which is suggested by this framework is the payment of informal carers. Ungerson, in advocating this as a way forward, discusses the advantages and disadvantages solely in terms of the implications for women as carers, failing to consider what the implications are for those who are cared for (Ungerson, 1990). And Glendinning dismisses the disability movement's demand for resources to go directly to the person needing personal assistance, saying 'It is not appropriate for reasons of both principle and practicality, to consider a system whereby benefit is paid to the disabled person to enable her/him to pay an informal carer for the care s/he provides' (Glendinning, 1988, p. 139).

Glendinning and others reach this position – echoing that of the Carers' National Association – because they are still focusing on what they see to be an issue concerning women's economic independence: there is no consideration of economic independence being an issue for those who need help with the tasks of daily living, of the way that such economic independence would enable people to influence the quality of their lives, or of the way that it would diminish the vulnerability to abuse. There is no recognition that disabled people may see the right to choose who should provide them with assistance 'as potentially liberating not only for themselves but also for carers such as family members who feel bound by duty to look after parents, spouses or disabled children' (Keith, 1992, p. 172).

Unfortunately, therefore, in giving voice to the experience of informal carers – or rather in the particular way that this experience was represented – feminist research has further legitimised the denial of the human rights of older and disabled people. Moreover, this research has significantly failed to challenge the social and economic oppression experienced by informal carers because it has failed to challenge – and indeed has done much to reaffirm – the social construction of dependency of old and disabled people.

The failings of the feminist research and analysis on informal care must also be put in the context of the fact that the academic sociology community generally has failed to develop a sociology of disability or of old age – instead both are conditions identified in the context of the problems they pose for society, for government, for other people (see Fennell *et al.*, 1988, pp. 172–3). Disabled and older people are treated as social policy issues and there has been very little challenging of the public attitudes which are held on impairment and old age, and a significant failure to explore the experiences in terms of the subjective reality of those who are old and/or disabled.

Conclusion

Both the public representation of carers as a pressure group and the feminist research which attempted to articulate their interests have failed to confront the fact that informal carers only exist as an oppressed social group because older and disabled people experience social, economic and political oppression. The consequences of old age and impairment include a high risk of poverty, a disabling experience of services, housing and environment, and the general undermining of human and civil rights by the prejudical attitudes which are held about old age and impairment. These are the factors which create a dependence on unpaid assistance within the family. The sexual division of labour within society in general and the family in particular explains why it is that two-thirds of informal carers are women; it does not explain why the role exists in the first place.

By taking the need for care for granted and by assuming the dependency of older and disabled people, feminist research and carers as a pressure group have not only failed to address the interests of older and disabled people but they have, unwittingly, colluded with both the creation of dependency and the state's reluctance to tackle the social and economic factors which disable people. In so doing they have failed to challenge either the poverty of older and disabled people, or the discrimination and the social prejudice which characterises their interaction with individuals and social institutions.

Part II
Independent Lives? The Experience of Getting Help with Daily Living Tasks

Introduction to Part II

The following five chapters explore the experiences of fifty people, whose ages range between 19 and 55, all of whom need physical help in going about their daily lives. The intention is to further an understanding of what it is like to receive personal assistance in a variety of different forms – in a residential setting, from family members, from statutory services and from paid assistants. Chapter 6 explores how people who need personal assistance can also be care-givers, a role which is very rarely recognised but which was the experience of a fifth of the sample.

The fifty people interviewed lived in one of four different parts of England, which included north and south, inner city, town and rural areas. Contacts were made through social services area teams, independent living projects, organisations of and for disabled people. The sample covered a wide range of situations, the common factor being that people required at least some personal assistance in their daily lives. Additional sampling was carried out to ensure that black and ethnic minority people and gay men and lesbians were properly represented.

All interviews were carried out with the disabled person on his/her own, with one exception where a personal assistant interpreted for a man with a significant speech impairment. This obviously was not ideal but subsequent written communication was established with this man as he had independent access to a word processor. Five other people had significant speech impairments but the researcher was able to understand them.

After each interview a typed transcript was sent to the interviewee with the opportunity to comment on this at a subsequent interview or in writing. Thirty-six people were interviewed a second time face to face; telephone interviews were carried out with six others, four people gave their written responses to the transcript and to further questions, and it was not possible to interview the remaining four, for a variety of reasons.

A number of people were very concerned that their anonymity should be preserved. Pseudonyms are used for all interviewees but, for some, additional care has been taken to ensure that they cannot be identified. Such assurance was vital to enable people to share experiences which were often very painful.

4

The experience of residential care

Very little has been written on the experience of residential care from the point of view of people living in such places. What is it like to share helpers with a number of other people? What is it like to live with people with whom you would not necessarily choose to live? Do people in residential establishments feel isolated and dependent? Or do they feel secure in the knowledge that help is available 24 hours a day, 7 days a week? Why do people enter residential care? Do they want to stay there or are they desperate for a home of their own?

There were various answers to these questions amongst the total of twenty-one people interviewed who had experience of residential care, ten of whom were still in residential establishments. Some people felt they were made dependent by residential care, but others thought that they could achieve a high level of independence because help was available on a 24-hour basis. While a number of people experienced powerlessness, isolation and sometimes physical abuse, a few people experienced residential care as giving them a freedom which they could not have when living in their parents' home.

It was quite common for young disabled people to have entered residential care in an attempt to leave the parental home, while others did this because there was no other way that they could get the personal assistance they needed.

Choices and constraints

For some people who are born with an impairment or acquire one in childhood, their early lives are dominated by residential care and the only choices open to them as they enter adulthood concern the kind of residential establishment into which they should move. Patrick, for instance, spent most of his childhood and young adulthood in residential provision of one kind or another: hospital, a residential College, a Cheshire Home and then, when he was 21 years old, he moved into an establishment run by a voluntary organisation. He was keenly aware of his lack of choice at this point. 'When I first moved [there] I wanted to live independently because ... I can remember the day so well. I thought, well this was it. I felt the only way out of here now was in a box. I thought it was the end of my life, I really did.' Patrick explained that he went there 'because there was nowhere else. It was the best of a bad lot basically. I had nowhere else to live and I needed the care and support. But I made a promise to myself that I would do whatever I could to get out of there in two years – but it took six.'

Patrick was asked what was so awful about moving into the residential establishment. 'I think it's this feeling of dependency on other people. And again it goes back to this same old thing of routine. At that stage I was so hacked off at having my tea at 5 o'clock – you know, I'd had that for all my life – and my bath on a Wednesday. It seemed to be the same everywhere you go. And I couldn't cope with it. It just used to really wind me up.'

Patrick felt that he was being forced into a living situation which he would not choose but which was the only option open to him as he reached adulthood. Other people are forced into residential care when their family situation changes, as Philip was when his parents died. 'My mum died first and then some years later my father died. We hadn't made plans for what would happen. He was quite healthy but then he got a lung complaint and within a week he had died. So I had to go into hospital.' He was in his late thirties and he spent a year 'on a geriatric ward just looking for somewhere to go'. During that year he was conscious that he was choosing where he would be 'for years and years. I wanted it to be absolutely right'.

Some people seemingly chose to enter a residential establishment rather than stay in their parents' home, although such choices are actually made in the context of significant constraints. Some move into residential care because they feel there is no place for them in the community in which they live. Louise was 17 in 1962 when she 'chose' to enter a large institution. 'I had two older brothers and they were working and bringing in a wage but whenever I went for a job as soon as they knew I had epilepsy they treat you as if you've got two heads. I get on with my folks, still do, but it was really bugging me that I couldn't get a job. That my brothers were bringing money home and I wasn't. My mother didn't object to me being at home but I just felt like the black sheep in the family. I couldn't get a job and I felt really awful. I just wanted to go somewhere where there were other people with epilepsy but it was the biggest mistake of my life.'

She went on, 'My mother didn't believe that I was going to go, she thought it was a teenage prank. I just said to the woman behind the desk [in the Labour Exchange] I want to go away somewhere. I said there are places for blind or deaf people, there must be a place for people with epilepsy. She had all these phones on her desk and she made some phone calls, and then she said be ready in the morning an ambulance will come come for you.'

At 9 o'clock the next morning an ambulance took Louise to an institution for 'epileptics'. 'It was a really massive place, like a village. It had its own shop and laundry and morgue, its own picture hall and dance hall. It was very institutionalised – there were all dormitories, go like that and you could touch the next bed. There were lots of other teenagers and they would drop down like flies so if you had a fit no one would bat an eyelid. I will admit I did like it at first.' Louise was there for 23 years, experienced mental illness, was paralysed by a medical 'accident' and only moved out into a smaller residential establishment when this large institution was closed down.

Disabled young people often have difficulty in creating an independent life away from the parental home and, for some, a move into residential care seems the only way to establish such independence. Ian's education had suffered because of a refusal to allow him access to mainstream schooling and he reached the age of 16 with very few options open to him. 'They [his parents] tried to get me into the local school, it was just round the corner. My mum said she would push me there and bring me back for lunch and things like that but they said, no, they couldn't cater for me. So in the end they sent a little old lady who had already retired as a schoolteacher. She was lovely but she had never taught anybody over the age of 10 and she started teaching me when I was about 9 and I very quickly outstripped her with my need for knowledge and my need for learning. So I suppose really I was lucky enough to pick up books and read quite a lot.'

The denial of educational opportunities makes it difficult to achieve economic independence as a disabled adolescent reaches adulthood. The only way that Ian could achieve independence from his parents was to enter residential care. 'I was in that 15, 16-year-old age group where eveything to do with home seemed very limiting. And I think I was quite pleased with the thought that I was spreading my wings a bit.' He entered a Home for the Physically Handicapped, sharing a room with five other young men. He was there for 30 years.

Some people see residential care as a stepping-stone to independence. Jack felt that his only chance of establishing a life separate from his parents was to go into a residential establishment and then try to get a home of his own. He talked about the way living with his parents made him feel dependent. 'They only got a ramp to the front door when I was 18. I think that they just got so used to helping me in and out, you know when I was very small they had to and then as I got older they just carried on doing it. As a growing lad, it didn't do much for my ... you know, it didn't make me feel very good.' By the time he reached his early 20s, Jack was feeling increasingly frustrated by the lack of options in his life. 'I didn't think I would ever get a job and I really wanted to be independent of my parents. So I thought that moving into a Cheshire Home would at least give me a separate life ... you know, just in the sense of being somewhere else. But I did think, right from the beginning, that this would only be a stepping-stone. I had this idea that I would then get my own place – god knows how I thought I was going to do that but that was my goal anyway.' In 1985, two residential establishments and 10 years later, Jack finally got a home of his own.

Dependence and independence

People who sought independence through moving into residential care often found that they had merely exchanged one form of dependency for another. Linda put her name down on her local Council's housing list when she was 16 but in desperation moved into a Cheshire Home in 1985 when she was 20. 'I decided I wanted independence but it was a nursing home and it actually limited independence. Out of forty-four people only three were my age, the rest were aged in their 70s and 80s, but it was the only place I could find. I just got offered it through social services. Everything was done for you – you couldn't decide when to get up and go to bed.'

Philip, on the other hand, having assumed that residential care would make him more dependent, found that in fact it gave him more independence than when he was living with his parents. 'All those years I was living with my parents I had a fear of Homes, of places like this. I've always thought of them as institutions which most of them are, but the philosophy of this place is that you make your own home. And so I was wrong. I've found a place which is not an institution as such. It's a lovely place, it's my own room, my own home. If someone wants to come in here they have to knock. If I want to suddenly go out for the rest of the evening, I just say, right, I'm going out – I only have to tell them in case there's a fire and they need to know who's in and who's out. And there's no "when are you coming back?". It's up to me.'

Wendy also found that moving into a residential establishment made her feel more independent, but for her, unlike Philip who has no desire to move out, it has also acted as a stepping-stone to a home of her own. She first moved into a residential establishment in her early 20s where 'They helped me to get independent. When you went there every so many months they had a review and at my first review they decided that hopefully I would only be there for two years and after that I would move on to a bungalow or a flat with a friend.' But she went on to explain, 'That didn't work out because I had a lot of aggro from my mum. She felt that I wouldn't be able to cope in the community and she felt that I would just be dumped, she was worried that I wouldn't get any help. I didn't agree with her, I thought that I would have got help, but unfortunately the friend I was going to live with died.' Wendy then moved to another establishment which another friend had told her about. 'I wanted to come here because I liked the freedom that this place would give me. I could see that people wouldn't interfere with what you do, that you could come and go as you wish. I didn't want to be told that I had to be in at half past ten or things like that.' Within three years Wendy was engaged to be married and was then offered a bungalow, in the grounds of the residential establishment.

However, most people find that, once in residential care, it is extremely difficult to move out. Although it is now more common than it was for residential establishments to support people's wishes to live independently, there are major obstacles to moving out. Hilary found this when she moved into residential care in an attempt to leave home. 'I had wanted to leave home from when I was 18 years old but it wasn't until I was 29 that my social worker said she had some information about this place [and] would I like to come and try it. The idea is that people are here for a maximum of two years before moving into their own place, but most people are starting to go over two years because there's no suitable housing.'

Housing is a major barrier to moving out of residential care, but so too, sometimes, is the legacy of dependency on parents. Hilary had to contend with her own lack of confidence, created by the dependency on her parents who were, moreover, steadfastly opposed to her moving away from home. 'Living with my parents for so long made me more dependent than I needed to be. At home, because things weren't adapted I couldn't do much – I couldn't put the television on myself, or do any cooking. And I couldn't get in and out of the house at home on my own because there were steps and it couldn't be properly ramped because it was a tied cottage and the person who owned it didn't want a concrete ramp put down because it would have had to go in front of the garage. It came as a bit of a shock to my parents, they seemed to think I was going to go on living there for ever and ever. When I said I wanted to leave, there were arguments – they said things like "After all that we've done for you, we've looked after you and given you a roof over your head". And then it meant there would be less money coming in – because my benefits, the attendance allowance and the mobility allowance, wouldn't be coming in anymore.'

To live in a place where not only did she have her own bed-sitting room but there was a kitchen area off it and a bathroom attached, together with help when she needed it, created a feeling of independence for Hilary. 'The staff encouraged me to be more independent. We have set goals to work towards. Like, doing my own shopping, making my own bed. When you come here at first you don't know what to expect. You've got all this freedom to do what you want, it's a bit frightening at first. You can go out, spend as long as you like out, without my mother saying be back at 4 or whatever.' It wasn't until Hilary had been living in residential care for over eighteen months that she felt confident enough to take positive steps to get a home of her own.

Some people, wanting to assert their independence, find that the staff in residential establishments have certain notions of what independence is which sometimes come into conflict with their own. Jack, for example, had no wish to spend hours struggling to put his clothes on when he could be spending the time, in his opinion, more productively. 'They set these goals for you which they called "Independent Living Skills" but which were all about doing physical things for yourself. But really it's a total waste of time, I didn't want to spend hours putting my socks on when I could be at my computer or nattering with me mates. That wasn't *my* idea of independence.' Jack experienced a lot of conflict with the staff over his and their differing interpretations of 'independence' and he eventually moved to another establishment which worked to the philosophy of residents directing the assistance they required. But here too, there was conflict over what 'independence' meant. 'They said that if I wanted a cup of tea, I had to go into the kitchen with the member of staff and direct them in making it. And that was supposed to be about me having control over my life. Bullshit. I wanted to spend my time writing letters and making phone calls trying to get a home of my own and a care package – and if I wanted a cup of tea while I was doing that, why did I have to go into the kitchen and say, now put the kettle on, put the tea-bag in the cup, pour the milk in ... they were imposing their ideas on me again. I mean *I* couldn't make the cup of tea so why couldn't I just ask someone to make it for me? I wasn't asking them to write my letters for me because I could do that myself.'

Some people who have been in residential care feel that the availability of staff gives them a sense of independence which is difficult to duplicate in a situation where they are living in their own home but rely on family and/or local authority services. Susan looks back on her time in a residential establishment as a time of freedom. She went there in her early twenties – 'I just wanted to leave home and become more independent. It was good because I didn't have to worry about what time I came in or when I went out. I wasn't keeping anyone up because they were there on duty anyway. When I was there, with 24-hour cover, it was the best time of my whole life. Not having to depend on anybody, not having to think that oh, if I go out I'm keeping someone up until I come back in. That 24-hour care, that was the only time I can honestly say I felt free. Really, really free. I could get up when I wanted, go out of the door when I wanted and if I didn't want to come in until 7, 8 o'clock the following morning I wasn't keeping any bugger up.' But that experience belonged to her youth. 'It's different now isn't it? Now I'm married with a kid. I may have liked the freedom of Yew House but I don't think I could have stuck there for the rest of my life, I'm not that type of person. You knew it was an institution but I didn't treat it like an institution, I treated it like an hotel.'

Privacy

Privacy is an important part of feeling independent, as Wendy explained. 'I feel that I am living independently now in a way in that I can come and go and I can do what I want to do, but I feel that everybody knows what you're doing. Like if you have a visitor everybody knows about it. But once I'm living over there in my bungalow they won't know who's coming or going. You need your privacy. If they come into my room they do have to knock but that's all the privacy you get.'

26-year old Fiona, describing the residential establishment where she has lived for the past four years, says that 'I think it's great here. You can sort of hide away if you want.' However, she too feels a lack of privacy, partly because she has to share a room with another resident but also because of staff practice. 'One thing I really hate is that they keep a cardex on you. They make notes about your mood every day and the staff talk too much about the residents. I found out that they keep a record of when your period is due but they don't do it for me any more because I found out and told them not to. They do say that you're allowed to look at what's on the cardex about you but they don't make it very possible to ask, so I've never asked. I make sure that I don't tell people much because although they say they keep it to themselves they don't. When the staff do a handover from the day shift to the night shift they talk about what's happened that day and they will discuss the residents. I've complained about it but there's not much you can do because it's just the kind of place it is ... I think the reviews are an invasion of privacy because they talk about everything that you do, I've got one next week and I'm dreading it.'

Some people were understanding of why staff discussed residents amongst themselves. Hilary was of the opinion that 'The staff do have to discuss the residents when they do handover. They have handover at 3 p.m. and if something's happened during the day they have to pass over information – like if I'm ill it'll be down in the book, Hilary's ill, pop in and see her. I think that's OK.' But for others the knowledge that staff talked about the most intimate parts of their lives was a major intrusion. John and Rose, a married couple who live in a residential establishment, are very concerned about staff talking to each other about residents, particularly as far as their sexual relationship is concerned. A number of single people also objected to the way that a lack of privacy inhibited sexual relationships. Stuart, who is 29 years old and moved into a residential establishment to get away from his parents' home, 'so that I could do what I like, come in when I like', says 'There can be a problem with privacy. You can't do a lot without someone finding out or knowing, especially if you're a couple – if you get what I mean.'

And when Jack fell in love with Moira, another resident, they felt, as Moira put it, 'as if the whole world was prying into the most intimate details of our lives, we had to account for everything we did, justify everything'.

Communal living

Living in a residential establishment means sharing meals and other parts of your life with people with whom you have not *chosen* to live. It also means that there are always other people around. Hilary felt that this was an advantage of communal living – 'If I want people to come in I can just leave the door wide open.' And although John found communal living difficult, his wife, Rose, said 'I enjoy the company, I feel it's important to get away from each other sometimes.'

Derek was planning to move out of residential care, but was worried about being isolated and lonely when he did. 'I want to be able to have social contact with other people if I choose and you can do that here. I can't use the telephone or drive, so I will have less access to other people in the outside world than I have in here.'

Fiona, on the other hand, resented having to live in a situation where she had little in common with most of the other residents. When first interviewed she was sharing a room with another woman with whom she had little in common. Fiona found that in recent years there had been an increasing number of residents with multiple physical and learning impairments and she found this difficult. 'I don't really have a lot in common with people here. I don't think it's necessarily interests in common, I think – some people here have difficulties with a lot of other things, learning or whatever. If it wasn't for Jackie, the girl I get on with, it would only be really Jake and Daniel that I get on with, and they're men. I get very lonely. I think deep down I'm quite a private person anyway and that doesn't help.'

Ian, who lived in one residential establishment for thirty years before he moved out when he was in his late 40s, had built up a strong social life which revolved around the Home. The changes that occurred there over the years prompted him to leave but he wanted to retain the social base that it gave him. 'It was never my intention when I moved away ... it was never my wish to leave the sort of social base that it makes and no wish to cut off from the friends that I've made there. I really got to the stage when I was feeling very frustrated with noise, and banging, and people's radios blaring on at 6 in the morning and going on until 1 or 2 o'clock the next morning. Night duty forever wandering about crashing and banging, things like that. I had just had enough. Also the residents were becoming more multiply handicapped, there were becoming more mentally handicapped people there and of course I quite like a peaceful life and I was finding that the continual upsets, rows, yelling and screaming that you get with a lot of people who are mentally handicapped – it's not their fault, don't get me wrong – but it was quite honestly getting me down a lot. So when this flat came up [around the corner] I thought, well, great, I've got the best of two worlds. I've got my own life if I want my own life, I've got my own quiet if I want my own quiet but I've also got the sort of social base that I can keep going to'.

Getting the help you need

Living in a residential establishment with its 24-hour cover means that in theory the help that people need is there whenever they want it. And indeed, some people felt liberated by this knowledge. In practice, however, each person has to fit in with other residents' needs and, in some establishments, there is insufficient provision made to cover for sickness, holidays and turnover amongst staff. All this means, first, that routines are established so that the provision of help can be planned in advance and, second, that waiting for a member of staff is a common experience in residential care. People had varying attitudes towards both the routine and the waiting.

John rages against both. 'The routine isn't under our control, you can't even choose when to get up in the morning ... We can't do things spontaneously, everything except going to the loo has to be booked in advance ... At times we have to wait for half an hour or more to get help to go to the loo. It makes me feel dependent and it feels awful – it's the way that help is provided that makes me feel awful.'

Richard, who is 19 years old and moved into residential care from a boarding school, also objects to the way help is provided. 'I ask when I want help – there's a buzzer – but it takes them half an hour to come. It's very frustrating. Also I get nagged here, I don't know what they want me to do, it's because I'm young. They treat me like a child. The staff aren't supposed to tell you what to do but they do.'

Malcolm, who now lives in his own flat employing his own personal assistants, objected to the way that the staff in the residential establishment where he used to live 'pushed God at me all the time. You had to say prayers before you ate and had to read the bible.' So it isn't just the practical aspects of the way help is given that people living in residential care sometimes find wanting; help can also be given in a way which is experienced as oppressive and inappropriate.

Some men living in residential care want personal assistance to be provided by male staff and this can cause problems because most staff are women. John said, 'I wish we had more male staff here, there are only two and it can be embarrassing at times.'

Stuart is resigned about having to wait for staff – 'You have to put up with it because there's not a lot you can do about it' – but was not prepared to put up with the way he was helped to eat at supper-times. 'At meal-times when they haven't got enough staff to feed everybody, it's a problem, and it started to happen every day. They thought it was alright for one care staff to feed more than one resident at a time. I don't agree because your food gets cold.' He suggested that three people (including himself) who needed help with eating should eat early, at 5.30 p.m.: 'It took a lot of hard work to get them to do this. I just suggested it to everybody and it caused a bit of an uproar. We all had a meeting about it ... it took about four months to sort out a solution.' Stuart would like to cook more often for himself – there is a kitchen area in his room – but can only do this when he gets help from his keyworker. 'I can't do this often – once every 3 months or so. She has to balance my request to cook with others' requests to go to the loo, which is obviously more important.'

When there is difficulty in getting help to do the basic activities of daily living, it is even more difficult to get help to do what are seen to be 'extras', such as going out. John and Rose find it difficult to go out and visit friends, 'There is a vehicle here that we can use but it's difficult to get a driver. Also going out is very difficult because of staff availability because we need help at the other end.'

Isolation

Contact with the world outside a residential establishment can be limited because of the restrictions on the personal assistance available. Fiona, for example, very much wants to get a job but 'I can't because I would need help with care and the staff aren't available to do that.' Instead, she is trying to get 'home work' such as typing. 'I wish I could get a job' she says. 'It would make me become a part of the outside world and not be so secluded in this small world. Even if I only got home work I would still have to communicate with the outside world and that would help.'

Like most people in residential care, Fiona's life is also curtailed by the small amount of money which she has – 'I only get £11.40 per week pocket money, plus my mobility allowance. It's not enough.'

Sometimes people find that a barrier builds up inside themselves which prevents them from going outside the residential establishment. Robin describes how this happened to him when he lived in a Young Disabled Unit. 'My friends would come and visit me ... it was like being back in hospital again really ... you know, to be visited, people would come to me. I tried going to them, at first, to their houses, or I made arrangements to go out to the cinema and that, but it was always too difficult. You couldn't get a driver for the van, and you know, even if you could you couldn't get them until the last minute, the suspense would kill me, not knowing whether I could go or not. So I made these arrangements less and less and then I found I didn't actually want to go out. I would think, oh it's so cold and windy. And I got paranoid at one point about people staring at me and knowing that I lived in a HOME. And you know I felt like a hot house plant that couldn't survive out there, that would get swept away ... '

Each time I visit a residential establishment there are one or two people sitting by the front door, looking out. I thought at first that they were waiting for someone but most do not seem to be. There is a feeling of separation from the world outside and it seems as if the nearest some people get to making contact with that world is sitting at the front door.

Powerlessness

Some people experienced residential care as being a mixture of dependence and independence: they did not have control over how and when help was provided but on the other hand for many residential care was a way of escaping dependency on parents and could be a stepping-stone to a home of one's own. For others, however, the lack of control created significant powerlessness.

Robin lived in a Young Disabled Unit for two years and found that other people's ideas about what he should and shouldn't do made his life very difficult there. 'They had these ideas that I had to get up at a certain time, go to bed at a certain time, even go to the toilet at a certain time. And they poked their noses into what I did. I was told that I could only stay there if I behaved myself. It was so difficult you know, I had to keep telling myself I'm an adult not a child – because that's how they treated me, but there was nothing I could do about it. In the end, I thought I've got to pretend that I'm going along with them, smile sweetly and everything, because otherwise they made my life hell.'

To receive physical help from someone who makes you feel powerless can be very frustrating and in some circumstances it can be extremely frightening. Jack described how 'there was this crazy bloke ... well, I say he was crazy, but actually he wasn't that much different from the rest of them, it's just that he went a bit further. If I had been waiting for ages for someone to answer the buzzer and he came and if I showed I was cross he would ... not every time, that was part of the problem, you never knew when he would flip ... he would get so violent. At first it was just words, but then he would use the help he was giving me to push and pull me about. Sometimes it was almost as if he was doing it as a joke, you know, he would laugh. And sometimes ... I would try not to look at his face it was quite frightening. And if he was undressing me, or washing me ... actually I only let him do that once, I'ld rather stink than let him near me ... but I had to get undressed and if he was the one on duty well there wasn't much I could do about it ... he would touch me, you know, take hold of my penis ... it was really weird because it was as if I wasn't there and it was difficult to say stop, because as far as he was concerned I wasn't there so I couldn't say anything.'

I asked Jack whether he had told anybody about this abuse. 'I should have, but you see I'd already complained about someone else, who'd hit me – *that* was in anger actually and wasn't nearly as bad – and they'd had an enquiry and my complaint hadn't been upheld and I got a telling off from the Head of Home and given to understand in no uncertain terms that I was a liar. So really ... I was terrified of him anyway.'

It was common for people who were in residential care to feel that they could not complain about staff behaviour. There was a general feeling of, as Moira put it, 'what's the point? They only think you're being difficult.' Wendy said, 'We're told that if we want to complain then we should go to Mrs B. [the head of the unit] but I haven't done that because I feel that I can't complain to her about individual members of staff. And, you know, I've been told that if you want to complain about somebody you have to complain there and then but sometimes Mrs B. isn't on duty ... but anyway there's no point in complaining because nothing would be done about it.'

Leaving residential care

Louise described spending her first night in her own home after 28 years in residential care. 'My first night here my friend stopped here with me. I wouldn't say I was frightened but it was strange. But the second night she had gone. And I had this wonderful feeling. I thought I can get up when I want, I can go to bed when I want. I can have a drink or something to eat when I want. That's what being independent means to me.' It also means that Louise now does part-time voluntary work for a disability advice and information organistion and in her spare time goes swimming, pot-holing and rock-climbing.

Louise was one of the few people interviewed who received significant help from a social worker to move out of residential care. Indeed, until her social worker said to her one day 'How would you like a home of your own?' Louise had kept this ambition entirely to herself as years of institutionalisation had given her little confidence. 'I had thought about it but I didn't think I would be able to manage ... I wanted to ... I wanted to get away from everybody but I didn't mention it to anyone.' Once she said yes, it took 8 months to find a one-bedroom council flat, and the social worker also organised visits from the home care service.

For most people, however, organising housing and personal assistance is very difficult and they received little help in doing this from social services professionals. Patrick, having decided himself that he wanted to live independently, did receive some encouragement from the deputy warden of the residential establishment who put him in touch with a key person in the independent living movement. This person had been invited to speak on a social work training day which the deputy warden had attended. 'He gave me a few ideas and gave me something to work on, putting together a care proposal and advising me on matters such as housing, and really acted as somebody who I could go back to when I encountered difficulties.'

Patrick explained the work that he had to do. 'I did a care proposal which was what my actual care needs were and what it would cost and how it should be funded and that. I came up with the idea of treating this place as an annexe of [the residential establishment]. I did that because it was the only way of doing it. I wouldn't choose to do it that way and with hindsight I wouldn't do it again but at the time I was desperate to get out.' Patrick found that the only way he could get funding for his personal assistance costs was to continue to receive Income Support for the cost of residential care, thus the idea of treating his own flat as an annexe of Part III accommodation.

As for housing, 'I applied in the normal manner to go on the housing list, knowing that I didn't have a hope in hell because in their eyes I was adequately housed. We went through the business of filling in the form and calculating my points and they said to me that I hadn't got a hope. But I just ... you know I used the argument that yes, although I was adequately housed but I had a certain amount of points because I was sharing a toilet with 18 other people. And I just hassled them. I wrote to them every month, rang them up and said why shouldn't I be housed. And eventually they came up with this. To be honest with you, I don't know why. It took about a year and a half. For a while they wouldn't entertain the idea but you know, it's a bit of who you know. I got to know someone who used to work for the Housing Department and that helped.'

However, Patrick was only offered a one-bedroom flat although he needed a live-in helper. 'They said they weren't in the business of housing carers, so I took this because I knew that if I didn't I'd still be there. I gave the bedroom to the carer and I slept in the lounge.' He then applied for a grant to build an extension and although it was, as he says, a 'nightmare' having to live there while the work was carried out, Patrick now has the two-bedroom flat he requires.

Malcolm was luckier in that his local council recognised his need for a two-bedroom property. He was also able to get funding for personal assistance from both the Independent Living Fund and his social services department. Like Patrick he received most support from other disabled people, this time through his local disability organisation. Malcolm was also relatively lucky in that it took a little over a year to get the housing he needed, unlike Dorothy who had to wait four years for her bungalow. The funding for Dorothy's personal assistance at first came totally from her social services department but she had to organise the recruitment and employment of her helpers herself with very little help. 'Before I left ... I had to start thinking about advertising and getting people before I moved out. The minute I knew I was moving I had to find my own helpers before I moved out ... Social Services weren't very supportive in that way, there's no organisation that you can call on, only the home helps which are no good for me because they're not here for very long. I mean that's the only thing that I don't think is very good that there's nothing you can call on if someone goes sick, it's all worry, there's no emergency cover, you can't get anything. They encourage you to want to live out in the community but they don't help you in that way. I had to find my own helpers by advertising, it wasn't easy. The first two I got didn't stay, you know it's a worry, really. I don't know why, they were only here a week, one of them, I don't know, perhaps they thought it wasn't what they wanted to do in the end.'

Dorothy found it very hard coping with the new role of being an employer at the same time as getting used to living on her own. 'I found it hard, it's very hard when you first do it. Coming here and having to get my own people to look after me, it's not easy. I wanted to move out but when I did move out I was sorry in one way because I had always been amongst a lot of people; they were always there if you needed them. I used to be on my own at night and I used to lie in bed and worry suppose the helper who's supposed to come and get me up in the morning doesn't come. There's nothing I can do to get anybody. It's a real worry'.

Leaving residential care can be a real liberation – in the way that Louise experienced it. But institutions create dependency and a fear of being on one's own and, as Dorothy found, this can make it difficult when first moving out – 'I felt so lonely after being protected and looked after for so many, many years.' However, Dorothy now relishes her independence as much as Louise. 'It's been so nice living my own life actually, myself. Because I've always had my life organised for me, all the time ... it's been wonderful being able to organise it for myself.'

Such independence is something that Robert aspires to. 'I've been here for 18 years and I've been trying to leave for 8. I don't have control over my life, it's a nothing life here, really. I'm 52 now, it's desperate really ... not having ... I just want ... you know ... if I could have my own flat.'

The next four chapters look at the experience of living in the community and at the varying ways in which people receive the personal assistance they need.

5

Receiving help within personal relationships

What is it like receiving assistance from those you love? What effect does it have on your relationships? How does it compare with receiving help from those who are paid to give it? These kinds of questions have not been asked by research on 'informal care' because the focus has been on those who give personal assistance rather than on those who receive it.

Human nature and relationships being what they are, there are no simple answers to these questions. While one person will say that receiving assistance within a personal relationship is to be avoided at all costs, another will feel that this is an ideal situation. A complex interaction of personalities and material circumstances will determine which it is.

Love, intimacy and personal assistance

Bob and Moira have very different experiences in terms of their physical requirements and life style. Their common experience however is of a relationship where the provision of personal assistance is an expression of love.

Bob describes what receiving personal assistance from his partner, Andrew, has meant for their relationship. 'When I'm in hospital the nurses do the kind of things that Andrew does for me but it's not the same ... it just feels different ... you know they're very good at it and kind and I can chat to them ... but with Andy it's different. It's very hard to explain but I think it's got a lot to do with knowing that we haven't got long together and that he can make me comfortable and feel alright ... It sounds soppy but really I think it's an expression of our love for each other ... you know it's the ultimate "being there for someone". And yes I feel guilty and we get cross with each other and it's absolutely ghastly sometimes but the bottom line is that he's there and that ... well, we're very lucky really.'

Bob thinks that his experience of needing assistance is influenced by the fact that he is dying but in fact Moira, who has needed personal assistance all her life feels much the same about the way that giving and receiving help can be an expression of love. 'I was terrible when I was a teenager and in a funny way I think that the physical help I got from Mum was like a piece of calm in the middle of all that turmoil. I mean, we could be having the most awful row and yet when she helped me onto the loo it would all go quiet. Maybe it was that she'd done it all those years with ... you know ... well, love I suppose ... so doing those physical things was associated with good things for us. And she was the best at doing it, the next best thing to doing it myself, well, it *was* like doing it myself. Because she cared as much as I would about doing it right.'

Of those people who received assistance from families or friends, most felt that they preferred help of the most intimate kind to be given by those with whom they had loving relationships, whether it was a partner or other family member. Jackie, in describing what were the positive things about receiving personal assistance from someone with whom one has a personal relationship, said, 'I think if you have a relationship with someone you do have a basic recognition of someone as a human being and that makes it alright, that's one of the things. Also there's a lot of trust there, a lot of knowledge and trust ... I think there's an absence of embarrassment, you know if you need help in the loo or the bath or around bed-time, you're not likely to be embarrassed with your partner. There's intimacy.'

Julie talked of how her preference for very personal help to be given by her partner or her sister was tied up with how she felt about her body. 'For me, it's a hang up about having hairy legs. It's silly isn't it, but I don't like people to know that I've got hairy legs. Once they do and they still love me then it's OK, so that's why it's alright with David [her partner] and my sister ... I've thought about it and that's what it is really. It's so, so silly ... The strange thing is that I'm much more able to accept having thin and strange-looking legs than

I am to accept having hairy legs. Because there's a really good explanation for why my legs are a funny shape but it's unwomanly to have hairy legs, however much my brain tells me that I shouldn't think that.'

Being helped to wash, dress, go to the toilet and so on, obviously involves close physical contact between two people but it does not necessarily result in intimacy. It is the love between two people which makes the 'caring' relationship an intimate one. This kind of intimacy can be very special and some people feel that the provision of personal assistance enhances a relationship, whether it be with a partner, family member or friend.

However, receiving assistance within a personal relationship can also stifle independence and lead to an emotionally damaging and physically dangerous situation, as we will see. There are complex interactions between the dynamics of personal relationships and wider social and economic factors and it is difficult to be precise about what it is which creates dependency within a relationship. The following section explores some experiences which illustrate some of the factors involved.

Dependence and independence

Some people, particularly those who as adults receive personal assistance from a parent, are made to feel dependent by the context in which the help is provided. A parent's natural wish to protect and look after his/her child can become an inhibiting restraint especially when the world outside the home provides little opportunity for independence and, indeed, can increase dependency.

Rosemary, now in her late thirties, had been educated at home, the most extreme form of segregated education and unlikely to give her many opportunities for independence from her parents. 'I went to an ordinary school for a time but it got to the stage where they wouldn't give me work at home and they didn't like me not going in and they didn't understand why I wasn't going in, because it was a high school and they were sort of high fliers. And the transport got a problem and then they sent a taxi but it would always come too early. The pain got bad and you didn't feel well and they didn't understand. So in the end they said you'd better have a home tutor. So I did from about the age of 12 until I was 16 ... I got two hours a day for three days a week. She was our form tutor and then she retired and they thought that would be a good job for her.' Such an education did not open many doors for Rosemary. She also found, like many disabled young people, that becoming an adult did not stop her parents being protective and discouraging her from going out of the house.

'Where we lived at the time was very isolated and there was no way I could at the time ... I couldn't actually get out. I don't think my mother was really interested in me doing that anyway. The trouble is my sister is eight years older than me. There's quite a generation gap and when she left home ... when she became independent perhaps things were different. She got married at about 20 and left home and I was left as the baby. I suppose I was quite shy and it's very difficult because people don't always take you for your age, they sort of ask you what school you go to.'

Over the years, however, Rosemary has gradually asserted her independence, until now the help which her mother gives her is not just an important background support to the work that Rosemary does for a disability organisation, but is also part of a reciprocal relationship. The reciprocity has at least in part been created by her parents' own increasing needs for help. 'My father's nearly 72 and my mother's 79 ... that can make life difficult because they've got their health problems. Mum helps me get up in the morning, helps me with things around the house, lifting heavy things ... and I go out and do the shopping. It's give and take ... I wouldn't like to think I was sitting around being waited on. I think my mother does appreciate the help I give her. I know that after I'm away this week [the interview took place while Rosemary was on holiday] it'll be, I'm glad you're home, I could do with this, I could do with that.'

Rosemary thinks that her acquisition of a three-wheel outdoor electric scooter made a major difference to her life and the nature of her relationship with her mother. 'I couldn't get out of the house before I had the scooter ... It made a huge difference to my life ... It was a big battle because Mum didn't really want me to have it, she didn't want me going out alone and there wasn't anywhere to put it, and I didn't have the money ... she wasn't keen on me going out, I think she thought I might be attacked. I think that was the first time I really stood up to her.'

'My mother got used to it once I got it. It's much the same about being independent [i.e. about leaving home], she says "oh, you're not going to be able to manage that". But now, I go to all these housing meetings and other meetings and as she gets older and she gets more incapable she realises it's going to be ... I haven't put pressure on her but I'm going to be on my own one day anyway. And of course she's going to need more and more help herself. She has accepted that I'm going but I don't know what the actual day of leaving's going to be like.'

Rosemary is working towards the day when she will no longer be dependent on her mother for personal assistance. She has gained confidence from being the local contact for a national disability organisation and has persuaded a housing association to build some bungalows suitable for disabled people, one of which she hopes to occupy. Her assertion of independence is however, entirely self-motivated; she has received no help from social services professionals and has had to build up her confidence in herself in the face of both her mother's protectiveness and the outside world's tendency to treat her as a child.

Kavita, who experiences a similar dependency on her family, cannot forsee any end to it. Kavita does not speak English and local health and social services have failed even to make contact with her.

'I get no help from social services. I only recently learnt about these type of services whilst going to the Asian People with Disabilities Alliance – where many people speak Gujerati.' Kavita lives with her sister and her sister's 13-year-old son. Her mother also comes round regularly to help out. None of the family knew of the existence of grants for adaptations – 'Someone at the temple said that there was no such grant or help given.' Kavita used to sleep on the floor in the living room, 'But my back got so painful that my sister had to have an extension to build a bedroom for me. I feel really guilty about this, that my sister had to spend so much money doing this for me. She is a single parent and is financially struggling. We did not know where to get advice and information from. My health got so bad that they borrowed money for the extension but despite spending a lot of money, the extension is not sufficient; my bedroom is too small ... I can't get my wheelchair in. There is still no ramp by the front door, I cannot climb up and down three big steps. Therefore I can't even leave the house on my own.'

Kavita's need for physical help is increased by the unsuitability of her surroundings and, although she tries to help her sister by doing things like chopping vegetables, she feels a burden on her family. 'Being dependent means that I am a burden on my sister and mother, like my sister has to get me into bed. I can't do this on my own. But if I have the right type of aids and adaptations, I can do little, little things for myself. I feel like a total burden, I feel helpless.'

Kavita's feelings of dependency are created by the circumstances in which she lives and in particular the lack of help from outside the family. Such dependency is not an inevitable result of her impairment.

Pankash, who at first thought he would have to live with his brother, gained confidence from going to a residential college and decided he wanted his own home. 'Living with my brother, it's not a good thing because you are always supported. They don't let you do anything, so you don't know what's going on around you. It's like with driving, if you are not driving you don't know where you are when you go out in a car but if you are driving you know where you are going. When you go on your own you realise what is the reality of the world.'

Pankash's family assumed that he would live with them. 'When I came back from college – they had already done a survey for the extension to my brother's house and how much it was going to cost – when I came back I realised that no, I had gone independent life in my College because whenever I am going back to College I feel I am going home. Because it gives you more independence, because you know you are the master. When you go into your own room you are the master, whatever you want to do you can do it. You can go here or you can go there. Because if you are in their house you have to look at other people's needs, consideration. Like here, if I come in at 2 in the morning no one is going to point a finger or say why did you come in at 2 in the morning. I come sometimes at 3 in the morning and if I want to eat food I can go into the kitchen and get my food and eat it. But if you are living with parents or family it's where've you been and so on. That's really crucial. So I went down to the Council and I got this house. It wasn't that easy . . . I got it in I think 10, 11 months.'

Now that Pankash has his own home he can appreciate the help that his family gives him because it aids rather than hinders his independence. 'My sister-in-law . . . you see I'm not far from my brother's . . . for the shopping I give them a list so they do my shopping and they've got a key so if I'm not in they will come and leave things. So it's quite supportive.'

Asserting independence can be particularly difficult, however, when the need for assistance is part of being ill. Bob said, 'It's very easy for Andy to take on this role of looking after me, well, I want him to look after me but ... it's hard to explain ... it's kind of ... it makes me feel guilty to say it ... but I want things to be on my terms ... well not totally on my terms because after all it's a relationship ... but I don't want him to hide things from me, or take decisions for me. And there was a time ... it was when I was feeling really awful, so tired and things ... and I think he just thought I didn't want to be bothered with what was going on ... so it was easy for him to slip into taking decisions ... well, it wasn't that he just took them 'cos you know he would say ... but it was clear that it wasn't *my* decision.'

Some people who received personal assistance from a partner talked about the need to maintain some independence within their relationship, while at the same time recognising the way that the giving of personal assistance was a positive part of their relationship.

Catherine explained how certain equipment gave her independence from having to rely on her partner, Robert. A van which she could drive from her electric wheelchair made a major difference in her life. 'I think there was about six months that we were living here before I got my van, so I was driving to work and someone would help me out of the car at work and someone would help me into the car at the end of the day. And I would come back here and Robert and I had actually negotiated that I wouldn't have somebody in between 5 and 7 because there was one woman who was doing it and she went away and we decided we would try without it for a while.'

She explained why they took this decision. 'It was partly my not wanting to go through the whole interviewing thing again. It was also Robert's very strong tendency to deny the fact that I needed anybody else, you know, he would be able to do everything and there were no problems. I think he ... found it really difficult when he was here and I had somebody else here and he would try and ... if he was here he would say 'oh, don't worry I'll do that, I'll do that' ... Anyway we'd arranged that he would be back to help me out of the car, at 5 or 6 o'clock. And the amount of hours that I have spent sitting in the bloody car. I wouldn't sit in this road and I wouldn't drive into our driveway because I was too embarrased because I knew that neighbours would realise what had happened and they would either come out and ask to help or they'd just stare at me in pity. So I would always park around here and listen to Radio 4 *ad nauseam* until Robert came back. And he used to come back all full of excuses, 'it's been so busy at work' and 'oh god I'm sorry'. And I would be really angry becase he had let me down and if I got angry with him then he would get angrier. We talked about it after I got my van and both admitted how awful it was and he said how awful he felt. He was terrible at time-keeping anyway. But it was a nightmare. It was awful.'

It is also significant that Catherine was only in this situation of being dependent on Robert because of his feelings about her employing someone to give her the help she needed. She explained why she thought he found it so difficult to have someone else giving her personal assistance. ' ... it could be ... I mean sometimes I picked up from him that he was being quite protective and if he saw somebody ... a couple of times I've had helpers who haven't been very good at lifting and things like that and if he saw that going on then he'd get quite protective. But I don't think that was the overriding thing ... I think he thought he was the best, yes. I think he certainly had that. And that was important to him. I think it was important to me too'.

The availability of equipment and adaptations to a home can make a significant impact on the amount of help that someone needs and therefore the extent to which they have to rely on a partner, parent or other family member. Equipment and an accessible home (in the broadest sense of the word) can therefore create independence. However, the way that personal assistance is given can also create independence.

Moira's mother, for example, was willing to give personal assistance but determined to encourage her daughter to grow into an independent adult. 'I suppose I never really thought about the help my mother gave me when I was younger ... she was just there ... it must have been quite hard although she did fight hard to get other help and we did get some. But I never felt bad about asking her for help, maybe it's because it had always been like that, it was just part of our relationship. And we did get a lot of things that, you know as I got older, meant that there was more I could do for myself. She always said it was a good thing she was small because she could have the kitchen made suitable for me when I started wanting to cook and things, you know, it wasn't a big problem for her to lower some of the worktops and things.'

Moira's mother supported her in her wish to leave home and go into a residential establishment. 'I think she thought I was mad – well, I was but I wasn't to know what it would be like – but she said 'yes I could go but I could always come back if I wanted to'. But the biggest support she gave me was when Jack and I got together and then when I got pregnant ... she was brilliant then ... they all came down on us like a ton of bricks but my mum, well, it was her that really got us this place and helped us get the help we needed. And she was just round the corner and of course once Molly was born she was always here ... but then she would have been anyway, I mean she's Molly's grandmother but it was always good to have an extra pair of hands.'

Emotional damage and physical danger

Some people who are dependent on their families for assistance are living in situations which damage them emotionally. And for some an inadequate level of personal assistance can result not merely in a low quality of life but can also be life-threatening.

Elizabeth was at a residential school between the ages of 10 and 19. She was desperately homesick but was also very unhappy at home during the holidays. 'I come from a big family and no one helped me. It's more to do with being in an environment where you can't do things. They would argue over who had to help me. 'You do it; no, you do it, I did it last time'. Because there's nine of us there was a lot of "no, you do it". I needed a lot of help when I was living at home, I was almost totally dependent because the house wasn't adapted and I was more dependent because of that. If it was adapted at least a bit I probably wouldn't have been so dependent as I was. My sisters were growing up and wanted to do their own thing. Which is right isn't it, in a way. It was very hurtful though, you feel like you're nothing.'

This message that Elizabeth felt her family were giving her – that she was nothing – was part of the reason why she attempted suicide three times in her early 20s. 'The first one was the only genuine one, the other two were just anger' she says. But the suicide attempts at least got her some professional help. 'I didn't get any help from anyone else outside my family until I did my famous trick. That's when they all came. They always wait until the worst happens ... I got a social worker then. And when I did it *twice* in one year it *really* got to them! They started to think maybe there's something wrong ... That's when they recognised that I needed to move away from home and they got me this place [a council flat] in record time.'

Her independence from her family has improved her relationship with them considerably. 'At first my family didn't come [to visit] but after some time they came more and more. And now it's every week. Now they realise that I'm not a burden ... now they realise that I'm not dependent on them ... it's more on equal terms. I'm here in my own right and doing my own thing without them, without their support. It's much better because I'm not dependent. And I went to university and they had nothing to do with that.'

Like Elizabeth, Robin – who became disabled in his early 20s – also only had any contact with social services professionals as a result of an emergency. 'I was in a terrible state really. I didn't know what I was going to do with my life ... it seemed to be written off. My mother certainly thought that there was nothing ... that she was going to have to carry on caring for me and she hated it, I know she did. And I hated asking her, like she just stopped turning me at night or lifting me in the chair and you know we'd been told at the hospital that this had to be done but no one thought to ask whether she wanted to do it ... or whether I wanted her to do it. So I got these massive pressure sores and eventually got so ill with them that I had to be admitted as an emergency. And then the medical social worker talked to me about what was happening ... and that's how I got put into the YDU. It seemed like a liberation at the time ... well it was I suppose, for me *and* her.'

Both Elizabeth's and Robin's families – one a large Afro-Caribbean family, the other a white middle-class family with a mother who did not work outside the home and who had visited her son every day in hospital when he was first injured – seemed on the surface to be situations in which personal assistance would be provided. In reality, the level of assistance given was physically inadequate and emotionally damaging. Similarly, some people who received help from a partner did not get the assistance they needed and some experienced physical violence.

Audrey explained her difficulties with her husband. 'I've had multiple sclerosis for about 25 years, since I was 19. Not having a very good husband, in fact he's really rotten, I never bothered him with my disability. He didn't want anything to do with helping me, he didn't want to know.'

As Audrey's symptoms progressed she needed more help, especially when her two sons were still young, but she didn't get it from her husband. 'I tried hard to do everything myself and I didn't ask him for help. I didn't have a home help, I used to do all the shopping and cooking and housework myself, look after the children. I used to change nappies on the floor when I couldn't stand up. He didn't help at all – he used to bring me a stool to sit on so I could do the washing up. I wanted to leave for a long time but where can you go when you've got a specially built place which can accommodate a wheelchair and the council says you're housed. And where do you go when you've got young children and there's nowhere to go that's accessible. I wanted to leave particularly because MS accelerates with stress and I had a lot of stress. And I was tired out from the work ... it tired me out.'

Audrey started going into hospital for a fortnight every few months 'because I had to get away, I was so worn out. He treated me in such an awful way that the neighbours got in touch with social services and they came to see me.' As a result of this, Audrey was offered a one-bedroom housing association flat and was helped to apply for money from the Independent Living Fund. She left her sons, now in their late teens, with their father. 'I wanted to get away completely, I felt I had done my bit as a mother. I wanted to get away because my husband was making them a bit like he was. They didn't have any sympathy for my disability and didn't have any respect for me. I was just glad to get the hell out of it. But now they realise, now I have a better relationship with my sons.'

It was the existence of the Independent Living Fund which enabled Audrey to get the physical help she needed and thereby escape an abusive relationship. This was also the case for Paula who had been physically and sexually abused by her father for as long as she could remember. 'I can't talk about IT ... you know, capital letters IT and all that ... I know I should but there it is ... What I can tell you is how I got away, escaped ... I used to go to a day centre and we had a talk from a woman with a disability herself ... it was about welfare rights or something ... anyway, I got to know her and she told me about the ILF and she also put me in touch with the housing association that owns this place and so there we are, I made it. I'm very lucky really.'

Paula explained that she had never felt able to tell anyone what was going on within her family. 'My parents ... well, they were the ones that looked after me, didn't they? I didn't know anything else ... I mean it wasn't until I was about 16 that it suddenly struck me one day that I was going to grow up ... I suppose I always thought I wouldn't ... that I would die before then. I think my mother ... well, as I say, I can't talk about it ... But I did start to see on television, and once there was a radio programme ... you know, people who looked a bit like me and it occurred to me that well, it shouldn't be like this, that I could live differently.'

Although Paula had contact with health and social services professionals no one realised that her father was abusing her.

Vicky fell in love with a woman who worked at her residential college and they moved into a flat together, with Lorraine providing for all of Vicky's personal assistance except when local authority care attendants came in once or twice a week to help her getting up. 'It was hideous, it was awful ... obviously she was doing everything and the whole thing just went badly wrong. I don't think if you live with somebody that's your lover they should be there doing any of the personal care as well'.

Vicky was faced with the situation of being dependent on a very violent person for her personal assistance. 'Although at college, we used to have rows, the worst thing she would do was slap me on the face hard and I could cope with that. But then when we were in the isolation of the flat it became worse and physcially there was nothing I could do. The sort of pinnacle of that was when my brother left [he had called round to see Vicky] she came charging out of the room, grabbed hold of me, threw me onto the bed and shook me about, slapped me on the face and said 'don't you dare invite your friends round here again'. And then, you know, shook me on the bed from side to side. After that I was petrified to let anyone in the house. And you know I didn't. It was real bad.'

It soon became clear that Vicky's life was in danger. 'One night she was putting me to bed. When I lie on my back my arms are up by my ears, they don't lie flat at my side and I was just ... I have to have two pillows under my legs to be comfortable and while she was doing this she took up the pillow and held it over my face. And we weren't even having an argument. You know when you're passed that stage of holding your breath, it's past that stage of holding your breath, you know, when you would take a gasp of breath, it was past that stage. And when she took it off, I tried not to gasp, I just ... and there I was, she lifted it slightly and then she did it again hard. And then she took it off and carried on quite normally putting me to bed ... But a few days later I did ask her "why did you do that?" and she said "well, I thought that's what you wanted me to do because you're always complaining about the care attendants etc., I thought maybe that's what you wanted". And I said "well what stopped you?" and she said "I could see your hands wriggling." I said "well I want you to know that if ever I do feel like committing suicide I feel much happier if I do it myself or I'll ask you but please don't do it without me asking."

'I spent the next few days thinking "Christ I've got to get out of here", frightened out of my life, thinking I'm going to get killed. So I decided that was what I was going to do.'

Vicky used the local day centre as a way of escaping from the situation during the day and also managed to get more help from her local council's care-attendant scheme which was expanding at the time. She didn't feel able to tell her parents, who lived on the same estate, what was going on, neither did she tell anyone from social services. She finally managed to get alternative accommodation and personal assistance and was helped in this by another disabled woman from her local disability organisation. It took her over a year finally to leave as her initial attempts failed when Lorraine threatened suicide. 'When [the disability organisation] told me about the bedsit I kept saying "yes, I want it", "no, I don't". I talked to [a woman involved in the disability organisation] a bit about it all and she nagged me to go. Actually, when I left she got Dial-a-Ride to come and take me from my flat to the new one and she was in the Dial-a-Ride van which was really nice.'

Protecting loving relationships

Jackie lives with Ros and 2-year-old Dan. She is aware of the difficult balancing act that she and Ros have to cope with in order to preserve their relationship. 'With the personal assistance I get within my relationship, I think you have to be careful, there is a danger of becoming over-dependent and overly tied to each other and just not having any space and losing respect and losing interest in each other. And of the relationship potentially becoming quite abusive in both directions. If someone's over-tired and has been doing too much of the looking after of you they can get pretty pissed off and have a go at you. And equally if you're close to someone and they're doing a lot of things for you and they're doing them over and over again, it's easy for you to forget that they're a person. It's easy to forget that Ros is a person. If it goes too much. If there's quite a good balance in my life in terms of getting support and being able to do things in different ways and in different environments and stuff then it's really lovely to have Ros doing things for me because it's part of a loving relationship. But when it goes out of balance and it seems to be only Ros it's absolutely dreadful and you lose sight of the fact that we're lovers and that we're individuals and that we do actually love each other, because there's no space for it left. I think it's absolutely dire.'

Jackie spoke about the way that putting too much on Ros results in difficulties within their relationship. 'The thing is that Ros has had the main physical care of Dan on her hands and the declining physical ability of me. And the two have coincided more or less. So it's been quite a big thing really. And Dan has eczema which has really interrrupted his sleep. So Ros has been terribly, terribly tired. And that's the time when things go wrong between us because you know she reverts to her able-bodied behaviour. And I get really pissed off with her and we have terrible rows.' I asked Jackie what she meant by the term 'able-bodied behaviour'. 'Things that are exclusive of me or taking over. They're the two sins really aren't they? Taking you over and pushing you out.'

When a partner or relative is under pressure, respect for the disabled person's autonomy may be an early casualty of the situation. Jackie is also aware that her own reaction to stress can be hurtful for Ros. When talking about the issues raised by the need to tell someone giving personal assistance when they are doing it wrong, she said 'I think it's easier when people are really close to fall into a blaming thing and I think that's one of the things that makes it really bad when you're telling someone that they've done it wrong if you're blaming them for it at the same time. So the opposite of that is to manage to say things in a light non-blaming way or maybe even joke about them. But that requires a standard of perfection which I must say I fall short of, quite a lot of the time'. I asked Jackie whether she consciously tried to make it OK for the other person. 'I do when someone is doing it as a job ... I do it a lot less with Ros and that isn't good really because she gets undermined by it. I think I'm a lot less sort of deliberate with Ros these days because of the whole thing about me and her and Dan being so good together and my ability to have an OK relationship with Dan being so dependent on Ros and Ros being so unsupported herself and being so knackered. I mean it's a really unhealthy situation and I get really frustrated with things and I'm afraid I let it show.'

One of the major difficulties for Jackie and Ros is that there is no help available, apart from the help that Ros gives, to enable Jackie to look after Dan. 'The thing I was upset about is just the fact that we're so glued together. Like, my relationship with Dan is practically totally dependent on Ros so my ability to have separate time, a separate relationship with Dan is not there, and Ros's ability to have her own life is pretty non-existent as well.' Jackie has tried repeatedly to persuade her social services department to recognise this aspect of her need for personal assistance and when I interviewed her the second time she had just made another appointment to see the Care Organiser – 'I'm going to have another go, you know, to get someone for chunks of time to be there when I'm with Dan. I haven't got terribly high hopes about being successful but I do want to raise it again.'

Alan has also been engaged in a struggle with his social services department to get access to a level of help which would prevent too much of his personal assistance requirements being placed on his partner. Local authority care assistants and District Nurses assist him in the mornings but for the past 18 months he has had to contend with consistent attempts to cut back on the level of help given. 'There's definitely a feeling that Angela should do more. The thought that 'if she loves him, she'll do it all'. Those words were actually said by one carer – but to another carer ... Our relationship is jaded in one or two areas compared to what it was, that's because of the way we don't get the help we need, without any shadow of a doubt. The single thing which creates rows or an uncomfortable atmosphere between Angela and myself is the care.'

Alan and Angela tried to avoid both a situation where people coming in from outside imposed too much on their privacy and one where all Alan's personal assistance needs were placed on Angela.

They used to have someone coming in during the evening to provide help but stopped this: 'It was such a strain on the relationship. It was a balance between the extra help and the stress that having someone else around created. The balance fell in favour of doing without the extra stress.' At the same time, having someone else to provide personal assistance in the mornings means that Angela has time then for herself and also for the voluntary work that she does in a local charity shop. Alan says 'The fundamental request of mine, throughout all this, is that I want to remain independent, so that I'm not living on a razor's edge dependent on Angela all the time.'

While many people felt that the help they received from family members or a partner was 'the best', it was also clear that the kind of help received from those who were paid to give it had other advantages. For example, although Julie wanted to receive assistance from those she loved, it was important to her that she also received help from people who were paid to give that help. 'For intimate personal care I prefer my sister or David to anybody else but if it's for any other sort of care I would prefer social services because I'm more in control, more directing things.' She was also acutely aware of the way that having to rely on friends could disturb the balance of a friendship. 'I really dislike having to call on friends for anything really ... I mean it doesn't matter how often they say they don't mind it, I just resent the fact that I have to ask for it anyway. So I would always prefer somebody that's being paid for it, whether it's being paid for directly by me or by social services.'

Reciprocity was an issue for many people. In other words they wanted to feel – and some did feel – that they were giving something back in return for the help they received from family or friends. Moira was very proud that she had made her mother a grandmother and was keenly aware of how much this meant to her. 'Some of my friends don't have close relationships with their mothers and if they've got children I think that's such a pity because I know my mother has got such pleasure from Molly. When Molly was little I would look at my mother's face sometimes when she was playing with Molly and it would feel almost as if you know that I'd given her something, which no one else could give her.'

Robin described the difference between relying on his mother for personal assistance and relying on his wife. 'I get very involved with Laura's [his wife] work ... she knows she can bring it all home and dump it on me ... you know it's quite a stressful job and she's got a very difficult boss and sometimes she gets quite het-up about things... But I do like to feel that I can help her to look at it you know from a distance.' On the other hand, he thought that his relationship with his mother 'was all one-way. She didn't want anything off me ... there was nothing I could give her. But I needed her help just to survive each day.' Another significant difference in the two situations is that Robin depended on his mother for all his personal assistance whereas he now has other people who are paid to provide him with help.

The importance of receiving help from sources outside the family and personal relationships ran through many of the interviewees' experiences and was crucial in maintaining an equal relationship. Some people were very aware that, if their relationship was to survive, it was vital that they should not be dependent on their partner for all their personal assistance. In other cases, it was clear that relying totally on one person, whether it was a partner or parent, created an isolated powerlessness which could sometimes result in physical danger.

6

Disabled people as 'care-givers'

The majority of those interviewed felt that they provided some form of emotional support to those who gave them personal assistance, but there were also ten people (all women) who could be described as 'care-givers' themselves. Four of these looked after young children, two provided assistance to their husbands (one of whom had also looked after her mother) and four others provided support to elderly parents (and two of these had previously also cared for young children).

All the literature on 'informal carers' assumes that there is a clear dividing line between those who 'care' and those who are 'cared for'. This research project on the other hand illustrates that people who are commonly considered to be passive recipients of others' help can also be 'care-givers' themselves. The experiences reflected in the lives of the fifth of the sample who were 'care-givers' is so challenging of the stereotype of the helpless disabled person that it is of interest to describe just what kind of situations we are talking about. At the same time, it is possible to identify the factors which made such caring relationships possible and the barriers which created difficulties. Within these relationships, as much as within those already described in the previous two chapters, the issues of independence and dependence were of key importance.

Making it possible

Some people found it possible to give help in the way that they wanted to because they lived in a physical environment which suited their needs, they had access to transport and they received appropriate help themselves.

Naomi and Susan both have young children. Susan lives with her husband, mother and niece while Naomi lives on her own with her daughter. For both of them, access to physically suitable housing and to transport was the key to enabling them to look after their children. Naomi's husband threw her and her daughter out of their specially adapted flat and she went initially to her parents' house which was unsuitable for a wheelchair user and which therefore prevented her from looking after her daughter. Having presented as homeless to the (rural) local housing authority she was allocated a new bungalow. She says, 'It wasn't difficult getting this bungalow. It took three months from when I registered as homeless. They did offer me a place in a refuge but it wasn't accessible'. Once she moved into the bungalow Naomi did not need significant personal assistance herself and was able to look after her daughter.

Naomi is full of praise for her social worker who responded to her needs in a way which has enabled her to look after her daughter – 'He's been wonderful. Like I'm learning to drive but I've still got to get my daughter to the nursery school. So he arranged for someone to come and pick her up every day and bring her back. And they pay for it'. As she lives in a small village, and her daughter's school is 15 miles away, such support is absolutely vital. The only difficulty she currently experiences in terms of parenthood stems from the difficulties caused by her husband, whom she is in the process of divorcing. 'Every letter I get from his solicitor there's a complaint that I'm not looking after her. He took me to court for not looking after her. When I was living with my parents, he reported her to social services for being in danger. They came and saw us and said that she was perfectly happy. He tried to say that because I'm disabled I can't look after her. He wants custody of her'.

Susan was living in a residential establishment when she became pregnant. She and Tony got married and moved into a three-bedroomed council house after the baby was born, together with her mother and her niece (of whom her mother has custody).

Although the house had previously been adapted for a disabled tenant, many more alterations had to be made. The dining-room downstairs had been used as a bedroom but, as Susan says, 'when I had my little girl I said I wasn't going to sleep downstairs and her sleep upstairs'. A 70 per cent grant was given for a lift, 'closomat' toilet, shower and ramp to the front door but the kitchen, double glazing, central heating and patio in the garden all had to be paid for out of Susan's thalidomide compensation.

Susan was not able to provide physical care for her daughter when she was a baby and toddler and her mother provided this. This was one reason why Susan found herself a full-time job at that time – 'It was very difficult watching my mother doing the things I should have been doing.' Now that her daughter is 5 and Susan can do things like take her to school, using her electric outdoor wheelchair, she can be more involved in looking after her daughter and she has stopped work.

When people have control over the way that personal assistance is given they are able to become care-givers themselves if they so choose. As being a woman in our society is so tied up with care-giving, the ability to use personal assistance in this way is obviously very important to many disabled women. For example, because the help she needed herself was available it was possible for Rachel to look after her mother when she had a stroke. 'My mother died two and a half years ago and if it hadn't been for volunteers I wouldn't have been able to enable her to live at home for as long as she did. Due to her stroke she became disabled herself and I had to keep a continual eye on her, make sure her bills were paid, her washing was done. Occasionally if the home help didn't turn up, or meals on wheels didn't turn up I had to prepare her meals for her and so on. She needed a lot of prompting and reminding that certain things had to be done and some days she would be more confused than others and then when the help she needed became more physical there is no way I could have carried on helping her without the volunteers. She would have had to stay in hospital if I hadn't had the volunteers whereas after her last stroke she was able to come out and she lived for another 4 months at home'

Lauren is a single parent and has been able both to bring up her son and now to look after her mother because she employs personal assistants. Moira also employs helpers and emphasises the importance of being able to direct her personal assistance in a way which enabled her to be her daughter's primary care-giver. 'I first got PAs when Molly was very small ... I didn't want my mother doing the things that I would have done ... I didn't want Molly running to her instead of to me and it would have been difficult for her to stop that happening if at the same time she was going to have a normal relationship as a grandmother to Molly. So that's when I got the money off the Council to employ people and I could tell them exactly what to do ... you know, like if she fell over and hurt herself then they were to pick her up and put her on my lap so it was me that did the kissing better. And of course Molly was fond of my PAs but it was always clear that I was her mother.'

If a disabled mother is to look after her small child physically and not have to hand over this responsibility to someone else (in the way that Susan did when her daughter was a baby), it is necessary for her to be able to direct the personal assistance required. This is something that Catherine identified as an issue which had to be resolved in her relationship with her partner before they could contemplate having children. She described how Robert was not happy with having someone else being around to help her and went on, 'It's something that always worried me and it worried me about our future. It worried me about if we ever had a child what on earth were we going to do about that because it would be a huge problem ... because I wouldn't have wanted him to have been ... I would have wanted somebody else to be involved as my assistant in looking after the child and I think Robert would have found that difficult. And for him to be providing me with most of my care and looking after a child just would have been a nightmare, it just wouldn't have worked.'

Jackie, who is parenting within a lesbian relationship, grapples with the difficulties caused by inadequate help to enable her to look after Dan. In the previous chapter, she described the difficulties that are caused by her partner, Ros, having to cope with both a child and Jackie's increasing need for help. However, the other dimension to the situation is the help that Jackie needs to establish and maintain her own relationship with Dan. She has enlisted the help of friends but with varying degrees of success. She described how one friend was willing to help but acted in such a way that her own relationship with Dan got in the way of Jackie's relationship with him. 'There was one time when I got so fed up with her that I stormed out of the room and then stormed back in and said if you're looking after Dan I'm going out. So I went off out and when I came back Dan was in bed and we actually talked about it. I realised that part of the problem was that I didn't trust her on the issue of supporting me as a disabled mother and not being a stupid, taking-over, able-bodied, not-a-brain-cell-in-the-head person.' Their talk helped, as Jackie went on to describe. 'Because she understands more she's worked out her own way of doing it which is more supportive of me. For example, there was one day when she came and we went into the bathroom and Dan wanted to play in the wash-hand basin. And she lifted him up onto a stool and supported him but me and him played so she enabled me to be with him rather than playing with him herself. And then when he wanted her to join in then we all played together. And when he got soaking wet and we came back down to change him, and I managed to think that when it got to changing him that I didn't just have to let her do it all even though I can't do it all myself.'

The creation of the need for care-giving

There are many situations in which people choose to be care-givers. Disabled people do not want to be denied a significant part of what it is to be a parent, and sometimes helping a partner or one's own parents is an important part of that relationship. However, some disabled people have to provide personal assistance to a partner or family member because alternative provision is inadequate or does not exist.

Mary, for example, finds that she has to help her husband get out of bed most mornings because the District Nursing service is unreliable. 'Sometimes they come so late that it's past the time when he wants to be up; he may have a meeting he needs to go to.' It can take her half an hour to help him get up. 'But what's that to me? I'm going nowhere.' She also fills in other gaps in statutory services: she and her husband receive meals-on-wheels seven days a week and a home carer cooks a meal for them on weekdays, so Mary cooks at weekends.

She feels that they need more help than they get and is particularly frustrated about the restrictions on what the home help is allowed to do: 'They're not supposed to climb up steps or do anything which involves lifting their hands over their heads.' This means that some of the things that she would like done, as part of running her home, cannot be done.

Rachel and her husband have lived in their own home together for 18 years and for the first eight years, Rachel provided most of the personal assistance that her husband, who is more disabled than herself, needed. Rachel's health suffered and they eventually managed to get some help from the local authority who set up a volunteer scheme to provide personal assistance. However, looking back, Rachel feels that there were also positive things about providing assistance for her husband. 'Although there were stresses and difficulties when I did Michael's care myself, when it took four or five hours to prepare a very simple meal and then feed Michael with it, and do the washing up, etc., it was a very special situation, in that it had to be done in order to survive. It means that I've experienced just Michael and myself being alone and we were very close. When we were in residential care we were under a microscope as the only married couple in a place geared for single people. When we first moved out we had a high degree of privacy, yet now, with the volunteers, to some extent we've lost that privacy.'

Nevertheless, getting outside help with Michael's personal care needs made a positive difference – 'It liberated our relationship quite a lot because Michael was no longer dependent on me for his personal care. So it became more normal.'

Rachel finds that she needs more help as she gets older but that, because Michael is more disabled than she is, his assistance needs come first. 'He does have priority when resources are stretched. It is usually me that will compromise but of course there is a limit to what I can do and since I haven't been very well I find it difficult. It can cause difficulties between me and Michael and I can understand how the volunteers can get to resent me, because he so clearly needs more help than me.'

In spite of Rachel's increasing need for personal assistance, the local authority who manages the provision of personal assistance to Rachel and Michael continues to assume that Rachel is able to help her husband at night, and this has caused major financial difficulties recently because Rachel has had a number of spells in hospital and agency staff have had to be employed to cover for her absence. 'I was phoned up by the hospital saying "you need to come in again – your bloodcount's very low" – this is one of the problems that keeps happening – and I was being hassled by [the social services officer] that supports our project by saying "when are you going to be out again, because we need to know how many nights you're going to need cover, you know, how much time Michael's going to need in the way of help because at that time we were short of volunteers" ... I felt quite resentful, I couldn't even afford to be ill because the department was counting its pennies.'

Barriers to care-giving

Rachel's life is made difficult by the local authority's wish to rely on her as a 'carer' but some disabled people have difficulty in getting this role recognised. Jackie has been completely unable to get help from her local authority to enable her to parent Dan or even to function as an ordinary member of her family unit. When she had a fall and was more or less confined to bed for a few weeks she could only get assistance with personal care tasks and not with any of the tasks which she performed as part of her contribution to her household. 'The thing that they didn't recognise at all – they recognised that I had a need to survive and they didn't think that Ros ought to give up her job in order to look after me, which is a blessing, at least she had the right to go to work ... it's quite upsetting talking about this really ... but they didn't accept that there were things that I did in the household that because I couldn't do them and because I couldn't look after myself as well, it was placing an inordinate strain on Ros and therefore part of what carers should do should be the things that I would have done, like the shopping, putting Dan's washing on and – I don't know – we worked out a great long list of domestic things.' But the local authority would only provide carers to come in for one hour a day, three days a week, when Ros was at work, to carry out tasks which were strictly related to personal care.

Jackie was very upset about this. 'There's never any consideration of disabled people being part of a household and contributing to a household. You're a unit, aren't you? Not entirely because you're an individual as well but there are household needs. I've not met anybody yet who's involved in these carers' services who is happy giving a service to a disabled person in a family context ... Presumably I could have had someone coming in to cook the evening meal if I was on my own but as I lived with Ros that was out of the question – but I would have been doing that as part of my contribution to the household. It's really annoying because it's very destructive of your relationships and it also perpetuates this thing that as a disabled person you're supposed to be on your own. You're not supposed to have any close human connections with anyone else.'

Other barriers which prevent or make it difficult for disabled people to be care-givers are associated with inappropriate housing

and inadequate access to equipment and transport. Whereas Naomi
and Susan are able to look after their daughters because they live in
accommodation which is suitable for their requirements and have
access to the necessary transport, Maeve is confronted with
inappropriate accommodation and restricted mobility opportunities. She lives in a three-bedroomed house but cannot manage
the stairs. She sleeps downstairs and so does her 9-year-old
daughter – 'I can't do the stairs at all now but she's just in here
with me and that's that.' Maeve's husband has left and her two
sons (aged 21 and 17) do not provide her with much help, although
the younger one receives the Invalid Care Allowance for supposedly
providing assistance to his mother. Maeve gets no help at all from
health or social services. She used to have a home help but 'I don't
get a home help at all now. The home help I had she went into
hospital herself so I haven't had one since then. My ironing in there
is just up to here.'

Maeve has been trying to get an electric wheelchair so that she
could take her daughter out and also take her to school, but has had
no success so far. 'An electric chair, now, that would make a
difference, obviously you would have so much more independence.
But nothing's happened about that ... I was at the MS Society only
last week, they have offered me a grant but it's not enough to pay for
one. It'd be great, it would be such a sense of independence.'

Dependence and independence

A variety of factors can prevent a disabled child growing into an
independent adult, as we saw in the last chapter. When the parents
on whom someone has been dependent for years then become
dependent themselves, a very difficult situation can result – particularly if there is no recognition by health and social services of the
competing needs within the family.

Tricia, a single woman in her fifties, spent some years looking
after her parents. Disabled from birth, she was in her late thirties by
the time she felt ready to leave home but 'that was about the time my
parents started to depend on me, both emotionally and physically. I
think they wanted to be needed. They got much more protective of
me as they got older. Because they had let me do things before, that
was how I got on really, but the older they got they seemed to live

through me. My father would be outside looking for me if I was late home. It was awful.'

Over the years, life became more and more difficult. 'Things got really bad after my mother's hip operation. She became very confused and my father was already confused. My mother got so she couldn't cook – she got very confused about the meals. So I had to have someone to cook on the days when I worked [she worked Mondays to Wednesdays]. We've always had a home help but towards the end we had the Independent Living Fund money and there was someone here more or less all the time. I couldn't leave them here alone. The ILF money wasn't enough so I had to pay for some of the care out of my own money. From Thursday to Sunday I was more or less coping with them on my own'.

Tricia described the years of living from crisis to crisis with never enough help to ease the situation for her and her parents. Then, 'the Christmas before last, my mother fell four times on Christmas Eve. She had a viral infection. I called the police to help because I couldn't lift her up. She had cystitis and she kept trying to get to the loo. She didn't remember that she could fall. We got someone from an agency on Christmas Day and Boxing Day and then I got in touch with my doctor and she went into hospital. My mother was a lot better by then but I was exhausted. The thing was, I couldn't really keep my Dad here on my own because he'd want to go and see her. I had to arrange to put him in a Home. It was after that that I got allocated a social worker and it was recognised that they should [both] go into a Home. But it was a very slow process. They got respite care and they didn't really want to go into a Home. When people visited they used to con them into thinking that they were a lot better than they were. It wasn't so much that pressure was put on me to keep them here but that nothing was being done.

'Things came to a head in June last year when my mum was rushed into hospital with gangrene in her foot. They took her foot off and there was no way she could come back home after that. Dad was in another hospital but he kept escaping. He assaulted the staff and broke windows. There were special locks there which were meant to be dementia-proof but he broke them. He would turn up here. It was so upsetting, I lost a stone in weight. I was carrying on with my job because it was my life-line, it was my salvation. One day they found him lying in the road. It was a cry for help. They took him into hospital and then after six weeks they wanted to send him home. They said he wasn't mentally ill and that he should be at home. But he needed 24-hour care.

'They sent him home. My sister brought him home at 4 p.m. and I was due at 5.30. A carer was due at 5 to cook a meal and my sister had thought he could be left for an hour, because she had to go and pick her children up from school. But she couldn't leave him. He couldn't keep still, he wanted to go outside, so she had to stay with him until the carer came. But the carer didn't want to be left with him. So I was left with him and I couldn't keep him in. The neighbours kept bringing him back in. It was getting dark and he went to the hospital over the road and told them there had been a break-in. So the police came. By this time I was getting a bit desperate and I rang my doctor. She said give him more sedatives and put the mortice lock on the door. So I did that. And he rang the Fire Brigade because he couldn't open the front door. They came and I told them what had happened. I went to bed but he only stayed in his bed for five minutes. He wandered from room to room all night long, making tea, he came into my bedroom demanding to be let out the front door. I think it was only because I was lying down that he didn't hit me. I felt safer lying down. But I did have to get up to check that he hadn't left the gas on. I didn't shut my eyes all night.

'I got in touch with social services the next morning and he was put into a private home. They were quite sure they could manage him but they discharged him after six days. When they said they were discharging him I told my sister "I'm sorry, Margaret, but I'm not staying at home. I'll find somewhere to stay." She said "That's alright you can stay here." The police rang me up at work and said "Can you come and let him in?" I said I would but that I wasn't staying. So that's what happened. I let him in and he was very distressed that I wasn't going to stay. I asked the police to stay and see me to my car. And then he caused absolute chaos here for about five days. He kept going over to the hospital across the road. They said they didn't know how he didn't get run over. Age Concern kept an eye on him but they kept finding the gas on. He drove the neighbours mad because he was out there shouting in the middle of the night. The only support provided was the home help because once my mother had gone into hospital the ILF money stopped because it was for her.

'The manager in social services was wonderful. He got in touch with everybody and called a meeting. I had decided to come home by then but my sister walked into the meeting. Whatever my sister said it helped a lot, because he was readmitted into hospital for a fortnight, "to calm the situation" they said. There was a case conference after that which I attended and I said that we both had a disability and by placing us together we were doubling our own respective disabilities. It wasn't as if I hadn't tried. They said that they would try and get a Home somewhere which could provide both the nursing care and the supervision.

'My mother died about a month later and my father was put into a new unit at a hospital which caters for people with Alzheimer's. I agree he really would have been better at home but he needed 24-hour care. The consultant had said that was what would happen, that my social worker would arrange it. But the social worker said "there is no 24-hour care". There's the home help service, and home care, and district nurses, but no 24-hour care. They arranged for meals-on-wheels for him, they arranged for the District Nurse to come and give him his medication. I think the home help got in once. He was never here. He got himself admitted into another home one night after the police picked him up. They took him there. When they found out who he was (he had been there for respite care), they couldn't get rid of him quick enough. They left messages on my answer phone saying "Tricia, come quickly we've got your father here."'

Sadly, Tricia's own quality of life only improved after her mother died and her father was admitted into permanent hospital care. A year later, when she was interviewed, Tricia felt liberated and independent, and was enjoying life in a way that she had never done before. However, the unhelpful attitude of some of the professionals with whom she had come into contact while looking after her parents still rankled and, in particular, she was outraged at a comment her GP made during one crisis. 'In desperation I phoned my GP and asked whether she could get my father into [a local hospital] and she said that he's not in the catchment area, number 1. Number 2 he wasn't suitable to go there and she concluded by saying "there's no room for him in my flat". And that made me very angry because the tone in which it was said, obviously she was being sarcastic and I'm very upset about that. She was saying that there was nothing she could do, I didn't know how to take it.'

A lack of outside help and her mother's increasing personal assistance needs are similarly inhibiting Bina's independence. Bina's personal care needs are met by her mother who herself increasingly needs help. 'She has diabetes and she has heart problems. She needs some care, some help with getting into and out of the bath. She is looking after me and I am looking after her.' Bina, who is 47 years old, is torn between, on the one hand, wanting to live independently, in housing which is properly adapted to her needs, away from her mother, and, on the other hand, the knowledge that her mother needs her. 'I'm very touchy with my mum. It's not that I don't want to be independent it's that if I leave her, what would happen to her? I get depressed about the difficult situation. I want to leave but on the other hand my mum needs me.'

Bina feels that it is because she is Asian that she worries so much about her mother – 'English people don't worry but Asian people do. The difference for me as an Asian disabled person is that I am under the pressure of family.' She finds that her life is being restricted by this worrying. 'It's very frustrating not being able to do things. I want to go to college. I started last week and I was thinking I can't do this. I was thinking that I can't leave my mother at home. I was worried about whether she was all right and if she was worried about me.'

Lauren is faced with a situation all too familiar to many women, whether they are disabled or not. Just as her son is becoming more independent – he is now 15 – Lauren's mother is coming to rely more and more on her daughter for help. Lauren has to juggle with her own personal assistance provision in order to give her mother the help she needs and is finding it increasingly difficult to leave her mother on her own. When asked whether she had requested her social services department to respond to her mother's needs, she replied, 'Yes but they won't. I mean, you know, I'm here. What I was trying to get was cover for the weekend because very often I want to take Tom [her son] out or just go out for the day, especially in the summer. Like go to Blackpool. It's very difficult ... I'm tied. And also just doing the shopping. I can't take her with me so I do it with my helper but I worry about her being left on her own. I can't just go out and wander around markets or anything because I have to worry about getting back.'

Caring for others, in the sense of giving emotional and physical support, is part of human relationships. The provision of personal assistance enables disabled people to participate in the kind of relationships – with all their dilemmas, joys and sorrows – that non-disabled people take for granted. Moira, having been able to use personal assistants to enable her to care for her daughter now provides support for her mother, who, aged 85, has moved in with her. 'There's not much physical help she needs, just someone there when she gets up and to help her you know, with stockings and things ... and she's not that steady on her feet so it's better if someone is just there for her. And that's what my PAs do – I tell them that's part of the job description because after all I would be doing it if I wasn't disabled myself.'

Moira, however, has control over the personal assistance she needs and how she uses that assistance because she employs her helpers with money she receives from her social services department and the Independent Living Fund. The next chapter, in looking at the experience of receiving assistance as a service from a statutory authority or voluntary organisation, examines whether such services enable disabled people to participate fully in personal relationships and in society generally.

7

Personal assistance and statutory services

There is very little written about the experience of using health and social services, or those run by a voluntary organisation, for help with daily living activities. How do these services fit in with people's lives? Or do service-users have to fit in with the assumptions and priorities of service providers? What kind of relationships are established with staff employed by health and social services authorities? These are the kind of questions which need to be addressed if community care policies are to make independent living possible.

Of the forty people in the sample who were not living in residential establishments, twenty-three received at least some personal assistance in the form of services provided by a Social Services Department. However, only five relied solely on these services for their personal assistance. The service received took the form of help with domestic tasks such as cleaning and shopping, and/or help with tasks which are commonly called 'personal care', such as getting up, dressing, washing, etc. The services went under various names – home helps, home care, care attendants, family aides, and so on.

Five people received personal assistance as a service from a non-statutory organisation, i.e. a voluntary organisation funded to provide helpers, but this was not the only form of personal assistance received by any of these people. Six received a service from their health authority's District Nursing Service but again each also received other forms of personal assistance. A number of people had previously received a service from district nurses but did so no longer.

Responsive services?

One of the clearest messages to come through from the experience of receiving personal assistance was the importance of this assistance being responsive to particular and changing requirements and situations. If people who relied on a service run by either a statutory or a voluntary organisation were to be independent, then that service had to be both appropriate for their particular requirements *and* able to respond to changes in those requirements.

The only service which was unreservedly praised by respondents was that run by a disability organisation which provided an on-call system of personal assistants. People using the scheme were allocated a certain number of hours per year which they could use as they wished. They could arrange for help in advance but the system was also able to respond to a request for assistance at very short notice. Tricia, for example, got help within half an hour when she had been unwell and needed someone to come round to cook her a meal. 'I wanted something to eat but there was no way that I could cook it ... And that simple meal seemed to just pick me up and put me on my feet again. So I think that was marvellous.' She has also used the system to get someone to do odd jobs around her flat and to accompany her to a chiropractor.

Marcia has used the service to call out people to get her out of bed, help her to the toilet, help her to have a shower. She had originally had home helps from the local authority but they stopped coming because, at that point, she only needed help with the housework and the home help service would no longer do house-work. Marcia's personal assistance needs increased quite rapidly during the last year and she was in danger of using up all her allocated hours from the on-call support scheme. The scheme's coordinator therefore arranged for her to get help from what the local authority now called its home care scheme. However, she says, 'the on-call support workers do what I ask them to do but the home care workers won't do the housework. And they won't do shopping.' Valerie has used the scheme whenever her system of volunteers has broken down, which has happened a lot recently. 'With a speech impediment it's very difficult to deal with a stranger when you're under pressure. So I've tended to use it quite a lot, I mean yesterday I used 8 hours because of shortage of volunteers.' She finds that she is usually able to get one of two workers who she feels happy with.

The most common source of personal assistance provided as a service, however, was the local authority social services department. Few people praised such a service or identified that it was able to respond to their particular or their changing needs. Amongst those few is Mark who receives a service fairly closely tailored to his needs. Mark's personal assistance requirements are met partly through employing someone using money from the Independent Living Fund and partly through the home help sent by his social services department. The home help does housework but also, on three days of the week, comes for just 10 minutes in the morning to tie up his shoe-laces as this is the one part of dressing which he cannot do himself. Anna and Matthew, on the other hand, had help from their local authority home care service twice a day, seven days a week. It was this help which had enabled them to move out of residential care into a flat of their own.

Anna and Matthew appreciate the way that the carers sit and chat; this is part of the increased social interaction with people that they now value as part of living in their own home. On the other hand, Pankash sees the local authority home care service he receives (and for which he pays) solely in terms of the practical help which he needs in order to get to work in the mornings. 'The support that I need is the most important thing . . . Because I am working at a full-time job so I need it in the morning, early morning. I go out by 8.30 so they must make sure they get here at 7. They get me ready. They help me have a bath, shower, whatever. Then I am getting ready while they clean or something. They do any cleaning to be done in the house, the bathroom or whatever; they do the ironing, cleaning in the kitchen, clean the counter or whatever . . . I insisted they must come every morning because I must have help in the morning, that's absolutely vital so that I can get ready and get to work in time. That's more important, to be on time. Because I call the taxi and I have to be ready.'

However, although the home care service can give Pankash the help he needs in the mornings – 'It works out very well' he says – the service is not sufficiently flexible to give him full independence at the other end of the day. 'Basically I don't ask for them to come in the evening because I have a hoist and I can manage for myself. I insisted because otherwise I wouldn't feel independent. If someone else comes in the evening and puts you to bed, they come at their time and so you have to go to bed at their time. If you want to go out and come in late, with a friend or whatever, it's not possible to come in at 2 in the morning, or midnight even. So that's what I insisted, I must have a hoist that I can manage myself so anytime I choose at night-time I can go to bed. That's more important.'

Some people had a positive experience of a social services department being able to respond to changing needs. For example, Susan, who receives help for 2 hours each morning from carers employed by her local social services department, found that she could get the extra help she needed when her husband had to go into hospital. She felt that her good relationship with the care organiser was important. 'I've got a reasonable relationship with [the care organiser], like she knows I'm not going to ask for anything I don't really need ... They're flexible – you know what I mean – as long as you're not demanding.'

Restrictive services

The general experience amongst those interviewed was of services which were not able to respond to either particular or changing requirements and that the restrictions on the level and type of service delivered in consequence created major restrictions on their lives.

Local authority services are not available to help people to do anything outside their own homes, or even to enable them to leave their homes. For example, while Bina has a home help to do housework she cannot get anyone to assist her with getting in and out of her car. The type of personal assistance which is provided is therefore very limited and is, it seems, becoming even more limited in terms of what service can be provided within the home.

Some people find that their local authority home care service will not do housework any more and will instead only do tasks which are defined as 'personal care'; some find that while they can get help with both housework and personal care, this has to be done by two different people. Alan has been grappling for the last year with changes which his local Social Services Department has instituted, in particular a decision that home carers will no longer do housework. Changes in the district nursing service have compounded the problems. Alan needs two people to lift him and, on alternate mornings, he needs help with emptying his bowels. District nurses used to visit every alternate day for this purpose, but on these mornings would also help with lifting and bathing. However, district nurses are now only allowed to do what are defined as 'nursing tasks' and for Alan this has been assessed as being confined to bowel management.

These changes, together with a new policy which meant that the home carers would not do housework, have resulted in considerable conflict. Alan explained, 'On one of the days that the carers come in, give me say a drink of tea and then put me on my side ready for the district nurse to do the bowel monitoring procedure. There is then an hour gap before they start again. Now during this hour gap they at first said they would allow the carers to do some of my ... the extra linen, washing, that was created by this routine, so that they didn't sit around twiddling their thumbs. But when push came to shove they said they couldn't do that so it meant they were actually sat in the lounge for an hour, or even longer on some occasions, just watching Angela doing the housework or whatever ... what we didn't like was that they expected the carers to just be able to sit in our lounge as if it was a cafe ... I mean it would have been a bearable situation if they had been permitted perhaps to do something constructive while they were here but they weren't prepared to let them do that and as such we said we would prefer them to be out of the house during that hour. And the response to that was "we can't have our carers walking the streets".'

As the district nurses will no longer help with lifting Alan, the home care service has to send an additional person at particular times to help in lifting. He said, 'It's not very satisfactory from my point of view because it involves more people walking through the door and, you know, you tend to get worn out by a load of different people you know coming in, going out, etc. etc. And at this time of year when there's holidays and things like that and it needs quite a lot of sorting out, who's going to be available, who isn't going to be available, it becomes a major part of your life just to organise, just to work out, who's going to be coming and who isn't. That never used to be the case, it used to be fairly straightforward, now it's complicated, and complicated needlessly.'

The general tendency for district nursing services to restrict help with bathing to situations where having a bath is deemed to be 'medically necessary' and therefore a 'nursing task' is also reflected in Mary's husband's experience. 'We had to go through this whole thing of getting the GP to say that he needed a bath for medical reasons. The thing is that the home help service wouldn't bath him, I can't help him in and out of the bath, so what would we have done? Luckily we've got a sympathetic GP and she produced this argument for why it was necessary – but really ... well, you know ... it's a bit of a joke.'

A number of people said that their home helps, who have often been renamed home carers, will now only do shopping and personal care tasks and will not do housework. William, for example, found that tasks associated with continence are given priority over domestic cleaning tasks. 'I've now got to the ridiculous situation where they'll go and get supplies for me from the chemist, and they'll come and empty my leg-bag, but they won't clean the floor. The thing is I can get the chemist to deliver things, or someone to collect them for me, but it's much more difficult to ask a friend to clean the floor for you – actually it's easier to ask a friend to empty my leg bag than clean the floor.'

William found that, in order to get help with washing his clothes, he had to argue that this need was created by incontinence. 'It's ridiculous. I need someone to put the dirty washing in the machine, take it out, put it in the tumble dryer, take it out and fold it up and put it away. Well, obviously I do, I can't do it myself. But in order to persuade them to do this I had to say that I had these needs for doing washing because I was incontinent. Talk about making you feel bad about yourself!'

'Fitting the client to the service'

Forcing people to medicalise their needs and/or only responding to needs for personal assistance which fit the priorities laid down by the health or social services authority, rather than the individual's priorities, are both examples of 'fitting the client to the service'. This, unfortunately, was all too common an experience amongst those interviewed.

When Catherine's relationship with her partner broke down and he moved out, she approached her local social services department for help with the personal assistance she required last thing at night and first thing in the morning, help which previously Robert had provided. For some years she had employed someone herself for the help that she needed for two hours when she got in from work each evening and was very happy with this arrangement. She described the response to her request for help, 'One issue that came up was that he[the social services officer] was saying "with our Family Aides, we could easily send people round during the day time for the 5–7 o'clock slot". And I said, "well, I don't want anyone then because I've got someone already who I got on with very well and I don't want to lose her and I'm prepared to pay for her" ... And he was saying "oh well, this might be difficult. If we're going to give you anything then that's the easiest time we could give you someone". And he was making me feel as if I should give up this person who I've formed a really good relationship with, in order to fit into their services, which I was really quite angry about.'

Elizabeth spoke eloquently about the way that the Family Aide service run by her local authority is not tailored towards her needs. 'I don't feel I have much control at all over the amount and kind of help I get. It's very difficult ... I have to walk on eggshells. Although they say they're open to ideas, nine times out of ten my ideas get rejected on the grounds that they haven't got time. You see they service about six other residents ... or it doesn't fit in with their own philosophy about how the service should run.'

When asked what she meant by this, she explained, 'For example, I had a confrontation with them when I returned from University last summer. I put it to them that when I got a job I would get more exhausted and I would want to have help in ways which I hadn't had before ... like feeding. Because when I'm tired my athetoid movements [which mean that her body shakes] become more uncontrollable and obviously feeding myself becomes even more of an effort. So I just said, "would you help me, say, on the day I had an interview and I wanted to conserve all my energy?" One of them said that was like regressing. They more or less implied that when I was at University and got support from Community Service Volunteers (CSVs) that I had become lazy. They were trying to make out that I was sort of trying to put one over. They just took it completely the wrong way.'

Elizabeth also had problems trying to get the Meals-on-Wheels service to respond to her changed situation once she got a part-time job. 'I wanted them to bring it to my workplace, which is only just across the road, but they said it wasn't on their route.' Elizabeth's request for a service to be delivered to her workplace was not compatible with the assumption that Meals-on-Wheels deliver a service to people in their own homes. In the end, the Home Care Organiser suggested that Meals-on-Wheels deliver two frozen meals for the days that Elizabeth is at work – 'So on Monday they give me one fresh meal and two frozen and I heat them up in the evenings.' Elizabeth also feels that the Family Aide service does not take account of her particular cultural needs as an Afro-Caribbean woman. 'One of the things that annoys me is that they don't take account of our different culture. Ideally I should be able to have a helper who can do my hair. I'm not being racist but white people generally don't know how to look after Afro hair ... Normally I have an extension but I've got it out at the moment ... But combing that is a problem because when it gets untidy I have to go to the hairdressers and pay a bomb just to have it combed ... or hope one of my sisters will come and do it in a plait.'

She identified other things 'about being black which affect how I need personal assistance. They only prepare snack meals and really that rules out any ethnic food. Also they don't understand my relationship with my family, now that is partly cultural, the way we interact. Partly.'

Osman, on the other hand, has an Asian home help who comes three times a week and cooks him Asian food. But Osman was the only one of the five Asian interviewees who had an Asian home help. Pankash, through his involvement in an Asian disability group, is very aware of how many Asian disabled people are losing out on getting any local authority services at all. He feels that he gets the service he does partly because he has, through his attendance at college, been able to fit in with white society. 'So I become like just one of them ... I mix with so many people and with language now I can communicate. So in my case it works out well with everybody and it should be the same with others but they are not still coming into the mainstream and they are losing out with services. Once they get there they will realise.'

The question may be asked, however, whether the services should not be adapted to meet particular cultural needs, delivered in a way which ensures that people in minority cultures obtain equal access to them. Why should someone become 'Westernised', fit into the dominant culture, in order to get access to services?

Black and Asian disabled people undoubtedly experience both direct and indirect racism in their relationship with service providers. Sometimes, however, it is difficult to untangle what is racism and what is just a generally inflexible service. Osman, for example, wanted to go to a Disability Resource Centre because he was lonely and bored at home on his own all day. However, he was told that he could only do this if he attended a class so he tried to enrol for a computer class but was told he couldn't because he didn't have the full use of all of his fingers. 'I phoned about going there but they said you can't do anything, you can't come in ... They said to me, you can't come in.' He tried to enlist the help of his social worker but without much success. 'I asked my social worker and she said to me "yes, you can't do any" ... I said "I'm depressed and I must go there. I just stay at home and I am depressed."' Subsequently, Osman was allocated an Asian social worker who speaks the same language as him and who seems to be responding to his needs more sympathetically.

The role of district nurses

Although a number of people interviewed had used the district nursing service at some time in the past, only six people currently received visits from district nurses (and two of these ceased to do so by the time of their second interview). Some people had had help with bathing or getting up and going to bed withdrawn because district nurses now only did what were defined as 'nursing tasks'.

For most people who had used, or still used, district nurses, 'nursing tasks' were those concerning bladder and/or bowel management. Some people felt very strongly that such tasks should be carried out by district nurses and definitely not by partners or family members. William said, 'When I lived at home it was really important to me that they came in and dealt with all of that and that I didn't have to rely on my mother. That would have been dreadful.' Others no longer used district nurses for help with manual bowel evacuations because they had found alternatives which suited them better. Jack had felt really liberated by discovering that something which had been defined as a nursing task in fact didn't need to be. 'I read something somewhere, I can't remember where it was, but it was a woman writing about training her helpers to do manuals and I was just, you know, gob-smacked. We'd always been told we had to get district nurses to do it, and even in [the residential establishment] they'd come in to do it, it wasn't something that the carers there did.' Jack found that he could do without district nurses but it took a while to persuade Moira, his wife, that she too could do this. 'There I was, I didn't have to hang around waiting for them to come ... you know, Mondays, Wednesdays, Fridays ... you could never tell what time they would come and it would always take ages ... well, of course it would because you know I realised that it was a routine that my body was being forced into whereas once I could decide when I would ... you know ... go to the toilet, it was all different. But Moira, well she took longer to realise that it was just that simple. I think she was scared really ... well, you know, it's understandable ... all those years of *nurses*.' It was only when Jack had dispensed with using district nurses that he could seek employment; up until then he had been unable to leave the house first thing in the morning on three days a week because of waiting for district nurses to come.

Robin stopped using district nurses for bowel evacuation when he discovered that he could use a suppository inserter. 'It still takes a long time and I have to have a strict routine but well, I'm not going anywhere and now I only need help with getting on and off the toilet.' However, Robin still receives a visit once a month from the district nurse, 'I think they were reluctant to ... well, she comes and checks my skin and things and keeps an eye on things. It feels OK ... she's a nice girl ... '

While a number of people had in the past depended on district nurses for an important part of their personal care, and some felt very strongly that they should not be dependent on partners or parents for such help, their general experience was that the way the service was delivered did not assist them in exerting control over their lives.

Advantages of using local authority services

Although most people had a number of criticisms of local authority services, a few also said there were advantages to an organisation taking on the responsibilities of recruitment, being an employer and arranging cover in the event of sickness, holidays, and so on.

Susan says that, although there were 'teething problems' when she first started using the local authority home care service, 'I'm happy with what I've got. And I don't think I would want to be involved in interviewing carers. You can't judge someone when you first meet them and if you make a mistake what do you do then, you're stuck.' Susan thinks that she gets on better with the home care service than some other disabled people who use it because, she says, she is more prepared to compromise. 'Me and [the Care Organiser] talk about what I want; we discuss. I don't expect. And I don't think that just because you're in a wheelchair you should demand things anyway. It's a two-way thing, I don't think it should just be one way. I don't think you should look on it that just because you're in a wheelchair the world owes you because the world don't owe you bugger all.'

Although Jackie hasn't been able to get the kind of assistance from her local authority home care service that she wants, she still feels that there are advantages to using such a service. For her, this is particularly linked to the importance of equal opportunity policies. 'Things like, they've gone through a very rigorous selection process, the council has policies, they have the resources to train people ... I mean if I lived in an authority that didn't have a policy of equal opportunities for lesbians, for example, I probably wouldn't feel that so strongly but I do. I find it a lot easier to be out about being a lesbian with a local authority employee than I do with somebody that I've employed myself. I know that it's part of their job description to provide equal opportunities to lesbians. It makes it a lot easier for me to be open about being Dan's parent.'

Jackie said that, as she needed just a few hours help per week, she would only be able to offer part-time work if she employed someone herself. 'I think if you don't need a lot of ... asking for a lot of help ... then you're back in this thing of offering people casual or part-time or not very satisfactory employment conditions.' Therefore, she feels, there is an advantage to receiving help from someone who is employed by an organisation which can offer people full-time work with reasonable working conditions.

Julie was pleasantly surprised when she started using her local authority home care service. When her personal assistance requirements changed and she needed more help, her sister and her sister's boyfriend were staying, sleeping on the floor, and they at first gave her the help she needed. 'Once I started having social services coming in it wasn't half as bad as I thought it would be ... I thought they would be much more muscling in and telling me what to do, taking over. And, though there was one woman who is like that, and there are some aspects of it which I don't like, because the service isn't

good enough, I don't know who is coming from one day to the next
... and that's not their fault, so I can't take it out on them ... but the
people that I do get, I really like them.' Julie had initially felt guilty
that her sister and boyfriend were still there when the home carers
started coming. 'I felt a little bit guilty in that there was still people
around in the house who could have provided me with support,
when they were coming in and I felt I had to explain to them that this
wouldn't always be the case ... they were both looking for jobs and
then they would move out and of course you can't say when that's
going to happen ... And one woman said, look it's nothing to do
with me, you need me here that's all I need to know.'

Relationships with health and social services staff

Although, like Julie, a few people had positive experiences in terms
of how paid carers related to them, the more common experience
was of difficulties in this relationship. Most people, even those who
were happy with the general service that they received from their
local authority, had stories to tell of home helps and home carers
behaving in ways which were patronising and insulting at best, and
at worst abusive.

Susan says that she has had problems with the attitudes of a few
of her carers. She described one incident and its repercussions. 'One
argued about the way my underwear was placed and in the end I
said "who's fucking wearing it, me or you?" She went and reported
it and [the Care Organiser] came and said "well, I believe you
weren't very nice" and I explained the situation and she said "well, I
can see why you said, it but did you have to put it as strongly as
that?" And I said "well, I couldn't have put it any politer because I'd
tried three times before that to put it politely and this person was
just like" ... She said "well, she's asked not to come back in here"
and I said "well, can you see me crying about it?"'

Vicky feels that she can't relate at all to the care assistants who get
her up in the morning. 'They are all homophobic but they don't
know anything about my life ... they're not the sort of people that I
... you know I've always known that these people are only in my flat
because they're here to get me up. Under normal circumstances, you
know, they wouldn't be in the house, because they're not the sort of
people that I ... I can't remember there ever being a care assistant

that I've thought I wouldn't mind making a social friend of. There *was* one who was the same age as me and then I discovered she was a Jehovah's Witness ... I'm very much aware that I have absolutely zero in common with them but I'm also aware that they have no influence in my life. No influence whatsoever.' Vicky only tolerates this situation because the majority of her personal assistance is provided by people whom she employs.

Some people find that their impairment makes others feel uncomfortable. Elizabeth describes how 'When I have a helper for the first time, I have noticed that they are very uneasy with me. Not every one of them but most of them.' She has, over the years, learnt to deal with this. 'I used to take on all their discomfort and then I feel uneasy and then I feel guilty about the fact that my presence makes other people uneasy. But in the last few years I've learnt to take the attitude that it's their problem and I'm not going to get high blood pressure just because they have a problem with treating me like a human being. So now I just leave them to get high blood pressure by themselves. Don't laugh. It's amazing. Because I don't become uneasy I've noticed they relax. I don't know why it took me so long to work it out but I just don't get het up I just think to myself here we go again. And I just watch them. It's quite entertaining. I just be myself and obviously you can only remain in that state for so long and it's not a comfortable state to go around in. When they realise I'm not going to bite them or anything they soon chill out.'

Elizabeth was asked whether the way that carers felt uneasy affected the quality of the assistance they gave her. 'Yes', she said, 'sometimes they're very patronising. They're overbearing and they want to do more than I actually need. They want to give help in a ... this is a hard word for me to say but I'm going to say it ... in a custodial sense rather than facilitate. It's a big difference. When you're being custodial you're ... well you're dictating aren't you, more or less, you're smothering a person's sense of independence.'

Alan described a fairly common element in the relationship with home helps or home carers provided by the local authority – namely the judgement as to whether a particular person is 'deserving' of a service or not. Such judgements are based on a complex range of factors, including how 'grateful' someone appears but also how well-off they are in material terms. When asked whether the care assistants expected him to say please and thank you, the question obviously touched a raw nerve for Alan. 'Absolutely, absolutely. I cannot ... it's incredible some of the things that have been said to me. I mean, you've seen my house, you know what it's like, I did get compensation but that was 18 years ago, that is now worthless. I exist on benefits, end of story, and what little bits I manage to earn but that doesn't amount to anything more than about £10 a week. But they sort of perceive me to be still loaded. It's a complete misconception.'

Alan feels that he doesn't fit into what he thinks is the stereotype of a disabled person. 'They seem to me to have more time for disabled people who are really on their uppers, you know the ones on a council estate with their house falling down, low income, etc. etc. Presumably because that gives them more of a lift, to feel more important, you know they have this image of themselves, making this tremendous magnanimous gesture, even though they are getting paid to do a job, they get more of a lift from doing say helping someone in dire circumstances rather than myself.'

Valerie finds that some of the volunteers sent by the voluntary organisation which manages her provision of personal assistance have a rather romantic notion of 'helping the disabled'. 'Some of them think there's some glorification in "looking after the disabled". And they only realise when they come here that it's bloody hard work ... It's difficult when you don't live up to their expectations. Some of them think that because you're disabled and need all this help that you're always on an even keel, you've got to be perfect.'

William has experienced a range of negative attitudes held by both home carers and district nurses, all resulting from the fact that – at a meeting to which he was not invited – his mother informed social services and health authority managers that he was gay. 'It took me a while to work out what was going on ... they were all so stand-offish but then one day, this woman just came out with a stream of incredibly vitriolic abuse. And then it took me more time to work out that they think that I've got AIDS – which I haven't.' William feels very powerless because he is dependent on the social services department and the district nursing service for the personal assistance he needs. 'I've tried talking to the home care organiser about the attitudes of her staff but she just denies it ... she says they get training and they just have a job to do ... but what can I do? I can't tell them not to come into my home, although I wish I could.'

William was one of three people interviewed who had been physically abused by home carers. He described being handled very roughly in spite of his requests for them to be gentler. 'It's difficult to call it as ... well ... abuse, really I suppose you would say. It's physical *and* verbal. It's just horrible, horrible ... difficult to talk about ... I put it out of me mind when it's not happening.'

Alan had been hit in the face by a care assistant when she objected to a joke that he had made when talking to his girlfriend. 'She took exception to the remark and clouted me across the face ... she wasn't joking, she was deadly serious. I don't think she meant to react as severely as she did. But I couldn't do anything about it. The following day when she came in I thought I'd give her a chance to talk about it but she just came in and said nothing about it. So I complained to the organiser ... but nothing happened. She had only been filling in temporarily anyway and I said I didn't want her coming in again. I was never told what happened.'

Michelle had been hit a number of times and handled very roughly by a home carer who insisted that she say 'please' and 'thank you' when requesting help. 'I suppose she was treating me like a child really ... I mean, they all did that but she just went a bit further.' Michelle did not have the confidence to complain – 'I can tell you I breathed a sigh of relief when she left. But really, maybe I should have complained because I heard that she went to work in an old people's home.'

Privacy

Interviewees were asked whether privacy was an issue for them. Some responded that they were so used to having no privacy that it no longer bothered them – 'I'm not being funny' said Susan, 'but my privacy has been invaded all my life.' Others, however, identified particular problems with the situation where personal assistance was provided as a service.

Elizabeth said 'We have the famous meeting which I'm not allowed to attend. Also generally when they come in you know they've been talking about you because one of them will say something and you haven't told them. They're always digging for information ... they always want to know where I'm going and I think they comment on how I live my life.'

Rachel described how she felt that, while some volunteers respected her and her husband's privacy, others did not. 'It's not to do with them being around all the time, it's whether you feel that they respect your belongings, your home. You soon find out what category they fall into. Obviously if you're working with a group of volunteers you can sometimes get a feeling that you have to be very careful about what you say because they're going to talk amongst themselves about you. There was one group of volunteers we had where we sensed that they were all so curious about us, about what we were doing, that it was difficult even to make a telephone call because we were afraid that we would say something that would pass on even more information.'

Robin and his wife had taken a decision to stop having local authority home carers and instead to pay for help themselves, partly because of a feeling that their privacy was not respected. Robin explained 'They just treated this house as if it were an institution and not as our home. Sometimes it was quite subtle, what they did, and it's difficult to explain ... it was like they had the right to do what they liked here and also that they had the right to do what they liked when they were doing the things they were employed to do ... you know, so we didn't feel we could tell them how to do things. I tried, but it didn't go down too well. It just felt such an invasion when they came in that front door, it was on their terms not ours.'

This decision to pay for help caused financial difficulties but Robin said that he and his wife both felt it was worth it – 'It was such a relief having nothing more to do with social services.'

Relationships with service managers

Some people's privacy had obviously been infringed by the way that service managers behaved, for example in the case of William, information about whose sexuality had been passed on to home carers and district nurses. Other experiences included, as we have seen, difficulties in getting service managers to respond to the type and level of personal assistance that people wanted.

A number of people felt that they had to behave in a certain way in order to persuade service managers of their need for a particular service. Marcia, for example, said 'I feel you just have to charm people, you don't get anything otherwise.' Michelle explained 'I don't want them to think that I'm being difficult because I don't think they'll treat me very well then.' This was partly why she didn't complain about the home carer who hit her. The other reason was that she had no idea how to go about complaining without making herself even more vulnerable. 'I've never really spoken to the organiser properly and I suppose that she would just check back with the carer if I complained.'

Some other people also felt there was a distance between themselves and those responsible for delivering the service they received. This distance added to their sense of insecurity when rumours were flying around about cuts in services. 'It's a bit disconcerting' said Elizabeth.

Others described the sense of hopelessness and helplessness that they experienced when trying to get access to local authority services. Maeve said, 'I suppose I'm a very private person and I hate having to beg for anything and it seems like me begging ... well that's the thing about home care, I don't want them to come in all the time, just to provide some help you know ... but when you ring and you're told, "oh, there's a big waiting list" ... I'm very depressed about it.'

Marcia described how she relied on someone from an organisation run by disabled people to help her resist a home-care organiser's suggestion that she should sit on a commode all day. 'It's difficult to say "no" yourself but she said "no, definitely not" ... so it helps having someone else supporting you.' Marcia does not lack confidence in other areas of her life but, like many people, finds it more difficult to assert her own needs. Rosemary, for example, only started campaigning for housing for disabled people in her area when her friend was forced into residential care as the only way of leaving home. And Tricia, who is employed as an advice worker, says 'I should know where to get help but it's difficult when it's for yourself.'

A number of people felt that social services managers assumed that family members, or even friends, would provide personal assistance and that this was used to restrict the service made available. Some of these experiences have already been explored under 'Protecting loving relationships' in Chapter 5. Elizabeth found that her family aides complained to their manager that they shouldn't give her help if she had a friend there. 'They got the manager and set her on me. And she really did go for me. I wrote her a stinking letter but she'd gone off sick ... she wrote to acknowledge my letter but didn't reply to it. She did say that I had brought up some interesting points ... I took their arguments apart bit by bit. It's really a dumb argument. You can't have human relationships because they're making me dependent.'

Minimal services, maximum dependency

A failure of statutory bodies to provide services which enable people to carry on their daily lives and engage in ordinary personal relationships can create a very poor quality of life and undermine human and civil rights.

Ibrahim, a 41-year-old man, is made dependent on his family by the failure of health or social services to offer him anything other than a very minimal service. He has a home help twice a week who does cleaning and the district nurses come three times a week to help him with emptying his bowels (they used to come every day). His father lives 15 minutes away and provides a considerable amount of personal assistance while other members of his family do his shopping and cooking. The district nurses come at unpredictable times – 'I can't say anything. What can I say?'. Ibrahim used to go to a community centre where he met other Asian disabled people but gave up because he was so often not ready when the transport arrived to pick him up. 'It's very difficult to get out, like I say, it's not just the transport – they send transport – it's getting up in the morning. My nurse sometimes comes 10, sometimes 11, sometimes 12, so if I say to transport I will be here 9 o'clock and I'm not ready, their journey's wasted. So I don't go ... So I just said leave it; I said forget it.'

Ibrahim describes the poor quality of life which results from a failure of social services managers to respond to the need for personal assistance. 'My father's helping me ... I don't feel very good about that, because you know he's an old man, retired, he's helping me and I like to give him a rest. But I haven't got any other help except him ... most of the time I open my bowels during the day when I'm in my wheelchair. Then I have to wait until night somebody come, you know these sorts of things you know.' Ibrahim's father comes three times a day to help him and has recently started staying overnight. Ibrahim is a widower – his wife died when their child was born – and his 14-year-old son lives with his family. 'I'm not very good about that but I see him mostly every day.' Not only is Ibrahim denied the opportunity to bring his son up himself but the lack of personal assistance services also means that when his father has to go away – as he has had to do twice in the past year – Ibrahim has had to go into hospital.

This kind of situation is an infringement of Ibrahim's personal liberty and a denial of his right to be a father to his son.

It is difficult to be positive about many aspects of the experience of receiving personal assistance in the form of a service from social or health authorities. Some people appreciate it when responsibility for organising and employing carers is taken on by a local authority but generally the picture is one of a failure to respond adequately to personal assistance requirements and real difficulties in the relationship between service-users and service-providers.

8

Paying for personal assistance

Eighteen people paid for at least some of the personal assistance they received but for eight of these this was combined with services from either a statutory authority or voluntary organisation and/or help from a relative, partner or friend. There were various sources of funding for paid personal assistants: own resources (earnings, benefits); Independent Living Fund (ILF); direct or indirect payment from the local authority; joint finance (i.e. budget administered by the health authority and the social services department). Most people used a combination of these.

This chapter starts by explaining the practicalities of paying for personal assistance, partly because information such as this – and, indeed, that contained in the rest of the chapter – is not easy to come by and will be of particular interest to those disabled people who are thinking about employing personal assistants. The information also raises specific issues for care managers who wish to help those who need personal assistance to achieve an independent living situation.

Setting it up

People generally found that information about the options available was hard to come by, delays were common when dealing with local authorities and the ILF, and more help was needed to get access to resources.

Each person using personal assistance has hidden costs which are not included in the assessments carried out by either the ILF or social services departments. These relate to the extra costs of having someone else in your home – food, for example – but also the extra costs of taking someone with you when you go out. And other, not so hidden, expenses may be incurred: the cost of advertising for helpers, employer's national insurance contributions, employer's liability and public liability insurance, the cost of covering for sickness and holidays of personal assistants, of training personal assistants, and of paying an accountant.

The only person whose funding took into account at least some of these costs was Lauren who had also successfully tackled the illegality of payments direct from a social services department (SSD) to an individual. Originally, when the SSD agreed to pay for Lauren's personal assistance, the money had been 'laundered' through a housing association. She was not very happy with this as it meant that the housing association, rather than herself, was the employer. A disabled friend advised her to set up a trust to which the money could be paid. As it is not a charitable trust Lauren herself, even though she is the sole beneficiary, can be a trustee. A solicitor drew up the Trust Deed and Lauren invited three friends to join her as trustees, all of whom have specific talents which are useful to her.

Lauren, who is in her fifties and has a teenage son, employs four personal assistants who are each paid an annual salary. She has someone with her at all times, including driving her to work and providing whatever assistance she needs during the day – from writing on flip-charts to personal care. She is also able to look after her 80-year-old mother who now lives with her. Accountability to the SSD is ensured by having a social worker on the trust (which meets every three to four months) and by the production of accounts. The total budget includes the cost of employer's national insurance contributions, public and employer's liability insurance, accountant's and solicitor's fees, and some allowance for advertising and expenses. The budget does not allow adequate resources to cover sickness and holidays and Lauren finds herself constantly juggling with asking her personal assistants to cover for each other.

Lauren is also unusual in that her local authority pays the entire cost of personal assistance. It is more common for a social services department to contribute towards these costs, the balance being paid by the ILF. Dorothy's SSD contributes towards the cost of her personal assistance requirements paying the money direct to her fortnightly (although technically, according to the Department of Health, they should not be doing this). Dorothy employs up to five people who, among them, provide 24-hour cover.

Other people had, like Dorothy, moved out of residential care because they were able to employ personal assistants. The most common source of advice and assistance in doing this was other disabled people and disability organisations.

Malcolm left residential care with the help of a local disability organisation which enabled him to get an ILF grant and a monthly direct payment from his SSD. He employs three people, one of whom works Monday, Tuesday, Wednesday nights and Thursday, Friday and Saturday during the day, another covers the days, Monday to Wednesday, and nights from Thursday to Saturday. The third person comes at 10 a.m on Sundays and stays until the following morning. In addition, Malcolm uses his attendance allowance to pay for four hours a week additional help with writing letters and so on.

Patrick, a single man in his thirties, spent most of his childhood and early adulthood in residential care but now employs one live-in and one part-time assistant. The hours are flexible and vary week to week according to what he is doing: 'We organise the hours mainly on a weekly basis. A lot of the time I go away, etc. so obviously my full-time carer will take me away and that ... Basically the full-time carer is working an 8-hour day, five days a week and gets time off in lieu.'

Some people find that funding is not sufficient to pay a competitive wage to personal assistants unless they are treated as self-employed. Moira and Jack, who are both disabled and who have a 7-year-old daughter, receive a combination of ILF and social services money which enables them to employ three personal assistants who, among them, provide 24-hour cover . When negotiating for funding, they raised the question of employer's costs – including the cost of recruiting, training new workers and employer's insurance – but were told that these costs would have to come out of the grant made. 'It's really difficult', said Moira, 'It would mean reducing the wage we pay them ... if we took everything into account, and I don't think we would get good workers around here for that money ... you know, there's a lot of competition from agencies and that, where they can earn more.'

Maria also treats her workers as self-employed. She pays for the cost of one live-in personal assistant and part-time help at week-ends from her own resources. 'I get industrial injury pension, invalidity, reduced earnings allowance – an allowance that I only found out

about four years ago. Unfortunately they wouldn't backdate it ...
they top up what you get now according to what they calculate you
would have been getting if you'd stayed in your job. But it was ten
years before I found out about it.'

She also says 'Nearly half my income goes out on care. The rest of
it goes mostly on the expenses of life for two – food for two,
entertainment for two ... I'm paying double all the time.'

Some people employed personal assistants on a more casual basis
because they only needed a few hours help and/or the help that they
needed varied from week to week. Wendy pays for an hour's help at
a time to enable her to get out of bed, help her around the house,
cook the dinner and so on, when her fiancé is out at work. He works
shifts so the times at which Wendy needs help are also irregular but
she has found someone who has a part time job as a cleaner and who
lives 10-minutes walk away and is therefore quite willing to be
flexible.

Robin and Laura had started off their marriage assuming that
Robin would only need help when Laura was at work. However,
Robin found that getting help from an outsider, even when Laura
was there, gave him a level of independence which enhanced their
relationship. The SSD would only provide help when his wife was at
work and, in any case, he wasn't happy with the type of assistance
provided so Robin and Laura decided to employ someone themselves. They find the workers they need through a students' hostel
close to their home. Currently, they employ two people whose hours
vary each week according to what Robin wants and when they are
available. 'They come round, usually on a Sunday evening, and we
sort out what suits them and what suits me. It works very well ... the
only problem really is the cost ... we can't really afford it but it does
make a huge difference.'

A comprehensive assessment of the costs of purchasing help was
not carried out, partly because of the hidden costs already mentioned, partly because comparisons would have been meaningless
because of the variations in the amount and type of assistance that
people needed. It was clear, however, that while the amount paid out
in wages varied between £41 000 per year and £6250 the variations in
costs were not always related to the amount of help purchased.
While, for some people – such as Malcolm – about £15 000 per year
purchased 24-hour assistance, for others – such as Audrey – a
reliance on agency staff meant that only a few hours help a day

could be purchased for the same amount of money. It is significant that while Malcolm had access to advice and support from other disabled people in organising his purchase of assistance, Audrey was dependent on the help of a social service professional who organised the use of an agency.

Before highlighting the way that employing personal assistants can increase the quality of life, therefore, it is important to stress that receiving cash to pay for help does not always lead to control over the way personal assistance is provided. Nor does it necessarily create a good quality of life. Osman's application to the ILF had been organised by a social worker who didn't speak his language and it is unclear what input Osman had in terms of being able to say what kind of help he wanted. He was assessed as only needing help between 8 p.m. and 8 a.m. and he therefore has little control over his life because he does not have the personal assistance which he needs during the day, apart from home helps and District Nurses who visit three times a week. He very much wants to be out of his home during the day but 'I just stay home and I am depressed and so, and so ... ' Yet other people in this sample have managed to purchase all the help they require for the same amount that Osman spends.

Independent lives

Although it is sometimes difficult to organise, the advantages of employing someone to give the assistance required when it is needed are enormous, and opportunities are thereby created which make a major difference to disabled people's lives. Where people did genuinely have control over personal assistance this enabled them to participate in social and personal relationships in the way that they wished – and in a way which wasn't possible for those who had to rely on services and/or 'informal carers'. Such control also enabled some people to carry on paid employment. Jack put it in simple terms: 'I'm a husband, a father and a breadwinner. And ten years ago I was in an institution where I couldn't even decide when I would go to the toilet ... you know, you can't really understand it if you haven't done it ... your whole life changes.'

Lauren has been able to bring up her son and to engage in paid employment because she has 24-hour personal assistance over which she has control. Moreover, this now enables her to have her mother, who is over 80, living with her and provide the help which she needs. Maria described how, when she interviews prospective personal assistants, she tells them 'you're leading my life ... It means I can get up in the morning when I want to, go to bed in the evening when I want to, go out when I want to, and lead the kind of life that I want to ... To not be reliant on my family and my friends ... to keep all that separate [so that] to them I'm me rather than someone who needs help.'

For a number of people who had experienced residential care, the contrast in life style was huge. As Patrick said, when I asked what the term 'independent living' meant to him, 'It means exercising choice and control, having the right to choose who gets me up and who puts me to bed. I have to be flexible. I'm involved in a number of different things, the Centre for Independent Living ... things like that, going out to meet friends. There isn't such a thing as an average week ... one week is very quiet, the next I'm in London three times ... it varies.'

Howard, a 38-year-old man who had lived in an institution for eight years, said 'Independent living means that I'm not in an institution, that I'm living on my own, living in the way I like. I can come and go as I like. I can be back at whatever time I like with no one having any say ... and I've got my own privacy.'

To Vicky, 'Independent living means that I employ people and basically that they are here to do the physical things that I can't do which allows me to have the life style that I choose. Basically when they're here they're here for me and not for them ... I recently did this tape/slide show course and I was the only disabled person on it. I could only do it because I employed people. Sometimes I was up until 3 a.m. in the morning preparing this slide show thing and there was no way I could have done that without ... even to get there every day ... I make sure that the people who work for me can all drive so there's no problem with getting from *a* to *b* [Vicky has an adapted van] ... I don't have to worry about physical limitations.'

Such experiences of independence, of participating in society on an equal basis, are far removed from the situation where a dependence on services means that people cannot go outside their own front door and where the level of help available is just sufficient to meet only the basic necessities of life. It is also important to recognise that control over personal assistance can create independence even when impairment is accompanied by poor health and a necessarily restricted life style. Robin, for example, whose health has suffered as a legacy of the problems he experienced when dependent on his mother for personal assistance, says, 'I don't think people understand that when you're ill it's even more important to have control over the help you get, when you get it and how they ... how someone does things. I always think I could cope with going into hospital if only I was well ... you know, I could be more insistent ... because they take control away from you immediately you enter a ward and if I've got a raging temperature it's very difficult to say no, I don't want that, or no can you do it this way. Whereas with the young women we employ ... well, they know that I have the right to say what they do and that's just accepted ... I have to admit really that I can't do much ... you know I've only got to go out on one day and it takes me two days to recover. But the point is that *I* decide what I do, and I couldn't do that when we had the care workers from social services.'

Robin is clear that, while he receives a lot of help from Laura, his wife, it is very important to both of them that she does not provide all the help he needs. Catherine, however, is grappling with her recent recognition that receiving help from a paid assistant is more important to her than it is to her partner, Robert. Their relationship had broken down for a few months and during this time she had discovered advantages in employing someone to help her with getting up in the morning and going to bed in that it gave her greater freedom and reliability. 'Another thing I've quite enjoyed' she said, 'is having another woman to help and do things like putting earrings in – which freaks Robert out – or trying my hair in a different way ... there are just some things he just can't do'.

When Robert returned and they both decided that they were committed to making their relationship work, Catherine found that while she wanted to continue to have at least some paid help in the mornings, 'he's reluctant to have a lot of input from someone else. It's quite flattering really – he's very pleased to be doing the helping again ... he's proud that he knows what to do and can do it. I have to watch myself, I have to let him know that others can do it as well ... We're trying to work all these things out at the moment. We've discussed about me needing help and about me enjoying more freedom when he wasn't around and what to do about that. We haven't come to a conclusion yet together but I'm thinking of asking the Council to pay for help three times a week, say Tuesdays to Thursdays so we have the long week-ends totally on our own ... The trouble with having people coming in is that we are at our most intimate last thing at night and first thing in the morning.'

Recruiting personal assistants

There were a number of different ways of recruiting personal assistants and people had varying opinions about what worked best for them. Howard – who employs someone for three hours a day – said, 'You won't believe this but I've never advertised. Because I've lived in this town for ages I've got to know so many people from my work in schools that when I did need someone I have so many friends and I just ask around. All the people I've employed so far have been personal friends ... There are advantages to employing personal friends as my helpers because I know them, I know I can trust them. With someone you get through an advertisement you don't know what they're going to be like before they start ... it is quite an advantage in that you at least know what you're getting.' Howard currently employs a mother and daughter who share the work on Mondays to Fridays, while a man who works in a factory during the week helps him at weekends.

Patrick's involvement in a Centre for Independent Living means that he uses an agency set up by the CIL to recruit personal assistants who mainly come from Scandinavia. He lives in an area where there are a lot of nursing homes and the competition from these pushes local wages up so he found it was a waste of time to advertise locally. The agency sends him application forms from people who are interested in working as a personal assistant – 'It's people who want time out, people who just want a change ... It's a bit difficult if they're in another country but I do talk to them on the phone and if they're in this country I ask them to come for an interview.' He also takes up references.

Apart from using this agency, Patrick often finds that the best way of recruiting is 'word of mouth' – putting the word out amongst other personal assistants users who may know of a suitable applicant. Patrick was asked how he assessed whether someone was going to be suitable. 'With great difficulty, but it's something I've learnt to do. I just get that feeling ... I'm not saying I've got it right every time. Sometimes ... it depends really on what I'm looking for ... if it's long-term I might have someone sitting in with me, friends or someone who's done it before, just someone to exchange ideas with afterwards.'

Lauren also trusts to her instinct when interviewing people. She usually advertises through her local Council's Jobs Update which is distributed throughout the community, in libraries, shops and so on. 'Some of it's gut feelings ... I'm looking for flexibility and now with my mother I'm also looking for people who like old people because if they don't it's no good for her.' Lauren echoes a number of other people when she says, 'I'm not looking for professional qualifications, nurses are definitely out. I'm looking for people who are enthusiastic ... obviously they've got to be strong and not have back problems.' Lauren would prefer that applicants didn't even have previous experience in this type of work, 'because I want to train them in my ways, right from lifting through to everything else. Because everyone needs individual lifting methods, everyone has their own way of doing things.'

Maria also said that she wasn't looking for someone with a lot of experience or qualifications. She generally advertises in *The Lady* for her live-in assistant and in the local paper for the part-time week-end helpers. 'I used to put in the ad. "young disabled lady" but now I put "active disabled lady" because I'm going to be 40 next month. I put "aged 25–35 preferred" because otherwise I get retired nurses replying who want to mother me.'

When applicants ring up Maria explains the basic tasks involved and then asks whether they have any experience. 'I don't particularly want them to have experience ... I'm just trying to find out whether they are super qualified, like being an SRN, because I don't want someone like that. I say to them, it's almost like sharing a flat with someone but you're doing most of the work.' At the interview she demonstrates a standing transfer with whoever is currently her personal assistant and then asks the applicant to put her back in her wheelchair. When I asked how she assessed whether someone was going to be suitable she said, 'I think it matters very much, in the first instance, whether people are quick to smile. Somebody who can be light about things. I don't know what it is really. I haven't gone wrong that often but I use my intuition ... and it also depends on how long they stay and chat ... it's very much assessing whether I can share my flat with this person.'

To people like Maria, the experience that they build up over the years of assessing a potential applicant is a more important factor in making a successful appointment than formal criteria such as references. However, their judgements are also based on their own self-confidence and self-esteem, something which some disabled people are lacking because of their previous experiences.

Robin, for example, had very low self-esteem as a result of being looked after by his mother and then his experience in a Young Disabled Unit. 'When I first interviewed people I suppose I found it difficult to imagine that I was really offering them anything ... it was difficult not to feel that they would be doing me a favour by taking the job. I don't think I was really aware of this at the time but now I approach the whole recruitment very differently and I realise now that I was almost, you know, apologetic, when I first started out. I mean, I didn't used to be so explicit about what kind of help I needed and that caused problems when they started and I had to ask them to do very personal things.'

And Moira said, 'My god, when Jack and I started out we hadn't got a clue. We thought we would need someone with experience and qualifications, you know, we had had it impressed on us so much in that place [the residential establishment where they both lived] that we were in danger of our lives ... you know that we needed this specialist care ... we started off with an agency and I think they were terrified ... you know two severely disabled people and a new-born baby ... they sent us nurses in uniform to begin with. Now, well, we feel that the less experience they have the better, cos, you know, *we* know what needs doing, *they* don't need to know, they just need to be told.'

Using agencies

Moira and Jack had started off using a private agency because they had been told by their social worker that this would be the best way of getting their personal assistance needs met. This was also the case for Mark, an African man in his late thirties, who was helped to apply for money from the ILF and then advised to use a local private agency by his social worker. He was relatively happy with this arrangement, one advantage being that when he was ill he was able to ask the agency to increase the amount of personal assistance that they provided. However, he did have difficulties with one agency worker and was reluctant to take this up with her: 'She started misbehaving to me so I asked [the agency] if there was anything I have done to upset her. I said if she has got annoyed she must let me know ... I had asked that she should do the laundry and ironing and when she came, for the first three weeks she did the laundry and the ironing but then she started just folding the clothes and not ironing them. I thought she was so nice so it was difficult for me to ask her about what she was trying to do. So I just left it for another four weeks and she was doing the same thing and I was worried and I phoned the Care Manager and mentioned it to her that if she could send me another care assistant because this lady had started misbehaving to me. So they did send me somebody else.'

After Mark was burgled he decided he did not want strangers in his house. 'When I was burgled I was so scared ... I was scared that someone would break into my house at night. I wanted someone whom I had known for a couple of years to help me.' He then started employing people from his local church.

Audrey was also told that using agency workers was the best way of meeting her needs. Her key worker, from an Independent Living Scheme run by the local social service department, asked her to specify exactly what help she needed and when. This resulted in agency hours being booked from 8 – 10 in the morning, 12.30 – 2 in the afternoon, 5 – 6 p.m. and then 10 – 11 at night.

The arrangement with the agency is that they send Audrey someone on a long-term basis. It immediately became clear that no one wanted to work such awkward hours so each time a new person starts with Audrey she negotiates with them. 'I state the hours, what it is, and they say well we couldn't possibly do that and I say well my carer who I used to have we agreed between us ... and it seems feasible to me that we can ... we just work the hours; they mustn't go over the hours. They come at 8 o'clock and we just put the hours together. So Monday, Wednesday and Thursday it's longer and it might be five and a half or six hours and we just take it from 8 o'clock and so she might go at 1.30, 2 o'clock. They just leave things, the kettle filled up and things, you know, to my requirements. So we just work it between us, it works out OK, you have to really.'

This means that Audrey is on her own, without any personal assistance available, during the afternoon and evening until another worker comes at 10 p.m. for an hour, to help her to bed. I asked her what she did about eating during that time. 'Normally my carer does me something before she leaves, but like today she's setting up the oven for me and I've got a pre-packed lasagne and she's set up the time and everything and I'll just have to be careful lifting it out, but normally she does it for me. She leaves me coffee in a cup and how many teas I want, you know, tea bags in the cup, and the kettle filled and the milk in the cup, all ready for my own requirements. And I can just about tip the kettle out. And she makes me a sandwich and leaves it in clingfilm, and the cat's other meal is left in the fridge as well.'

Audrey has mixed feelings about this arrangement. 'I like the space being on my own ... It's still better than residential care, really, it would drive me crazy ... the only thing I find difficult is that my feet spasm and come off the footrest and they're so heavy and I haven't got a lot of strength in me arms and I can be absolutely stuck somewhere, you know, say the phone rings and you're not near the phone, or the door goes, it can be a bit of a bind sometimes.'

Although Audrey pays the invoices sent by the agency with money which she receives from the ILF and her social services department, she has little control over how her personal assistance is provided. There have been occasions when agency staff have failed to respect her privacy and her home. 'One carer used to bring her husband on every shift and I had to say, "excuse me, can I have my medication now", and they were watching *Neighbours*. I went, "excuse me ..." And I couldn't stand it, she was such a bad carer ... she would put soap on and wipe it off on the towel and I went ... she said, we do it in the Home and I said, "not to me you don't". Another carer, who was a nurse working her days off with the agency, was reluctant to wash the kitchen floor. I asked her if she'd wash the floor and she looked at me as if it was foreign, alien to her. Some of them ... all they want to do is shopping, or sometimes just sitting down and drinking coffee and talking, they think that's it.'

Assistance from social services departments

Audrey had received help from her social services department in setting up her personal assistance arrangements but she was puzzled as to why she hadn't been encouraged to recruit helpers herself. 'I wish they'd ... I would have thought they had done that, let me recruit people myself, that's what my dad said to me, "it's a wonder you couldn't interview a few people".'

Eighteen years ago, when Maria was first paralysed, she needed help in re-organising her life. 'I didn't know where to ask or how to get it. Basically it broke up my relationship because the guy I was living with was doing all those caring jobs which he shouldn't have had to have done ... not that he ever objected to doing it but it changed the nature of our relationship totally. I think had I been secure with having someone to deal with all my day-to-day care there would have been room for us to have our relationship. I wouldn't have wanted social workers, OTs, District Nurses traipsing through my home telling me what I should be doing but I did need help in sorting out how to get my needs met.'

Maria had spent a long time in hospital and she identified the way that she had become dependent and how this made it difficult to regain an independent life. 'If you spend many months in an institution you're going to feel very safe there and when you come out people aren't at your beck and call. I felt I was totally out of control of my life ... I had no control whatsoever.'

She does feel, however, that help in getting personal assistance sorted out is best given by someone who has a personal experience of disability. 'I had two social workers who came to see me when I first moved here and all they did was talk and talk and talk and at the end of the day they could offer me nothing. I don't think anyone who has no personal experience of disability, either disabled themselves or has a friend or member of their family disabled, has any idea about my life at all.'

Over the past twenty years or so, a number of one-off arrangements have been negotiated with social services authorities where individuals have managed to persuade them to finance their personal assistance costs. There was usually no formal policy for enabling someone with significant personal assistance requirements to live outside residential care and individuals had to exert considerable pressure on social services departments. Lauren, for example, had to establish contact with the Chair of the Social Services Committee before the Assistant Director would even begin to discuss the kind of arrangement which Lauren was proposing.

Now that social services authorities are having to address, in the context of the community care legislation, the needs of an increasing number of people who have personal assistance requirements, there is often pressure to cut down on the costs of these *ad hoc* arrangements which have grown up over the years. This is Valerie's experience, and as this pressure has coincided with a deterioration in her health and a consequent increase in her need for assistance, she has felt under considerable strain over the past two years.

Valerie's social services department had, some years ago, set up a volunteer scheme to provide her with personal assistance. This meant that a voluntary organisation recruited 'volunteers' to work with Valerie, paying them a small sum each week and providing free accommodation. The cost of the scheme was funded by the social services department. During the period that Valerie's health deteriorated it also became more difficult to recruit volunteers – particularly during the spring and summer – and Valerie often had to resort to agency staff in order to meet her needs. This, of course, pushed up the cost to the local authority and a considerable amount of pressure was exerted on Valerie to reduce her personal assistance costs. 'At the time, I was working and if I was ever short [of volunteers] for whatever reason, she [the social services officer] would say, is it really necessary for you to go into work today? ... She said "in fact, what we'll do if the situation doesn't improve and you can't stop using the agency, and modify your life, we'll put you into hospital and you'll become a health responsibility".'

Valerie was eventually made redundant from her job and felt unable to apply for another because of the difficulties with her personal assistance arrangements. Finally, the social services department pressurised her into applying for money from the Independent Living Fund for agency staff at night, although she only needs help at night when she is not well. This money is now in fact used to subsidise the cost of running the volunteer scheme and for agency staff in an emergency, thus reducing the cost to the local authority.

Valerie is contemplating employing personal assistants rather than relying on a volunteer scheme and, in some ways, would like to be entirely independent of her social services authority. However, like other people she is aware of the disadvantages of 'letting social services off the hook'. As Alan – who is dependent on services and wants more control over his personal assistance – says, 'The ILF does have drawbacks because you don't have the back-up of an organisation. If you could stay with social services but have your own budget then it would be better because you would have the back-up of an organisation. I would like the social services department to employ the carers and the client would then have the budget to purchase the care as required.'

Maria also finds that there are drawbacks to her complete independence from service providers in that, in an emergency, she has only her own resources to fall back on. When first interviewed, she had just been let down by a new live-in personal assistant who had been due to start working for her. The costs of employing temporary assistants are signficant – as is the emotional trauma and the practical difficulties involved in finding such cover. Maria cannot afford to pay for agency staff, 'Agencies charge £24 for someone just to sleep in and if they're woken it costs even more. I think it's exploitative of people who really need help in order to survive in the community.' When she sought financial help from her local social services department for the extra costs incurred by having to find temporary cover, they would only contribute the cost of 16-hours agency cover over two weeks – and they then took five weeks to make the payment.

However, Maria does value her independence and control over her personal assistance arrangements and, like most people inter-viewed, would rather not be dependent on her social services department. As Jack says, 'The less I have to do with them the better. They see us as "clients", they don't understand our lives ... it's ... well, we've had nothing but hassle from those kind of people. We give them accounts once a year, showing how we've spent the money and that's it really, that's all I want off them is the money and we do our bit by spending it in the way it's intended for.'

Malcolm would rather all his personal assistance costs were met by the ILF so that he could sever his relationship with the social services department. He refers to 'interference by social workers' and says 'I don't get on with my social worker. At the beginning I made a couple of mistakes [in doing the wages for his personal assistants] and the social workers started interfering. I felt they were demolishing my plans, trying to take me over.'

Dorothy, on the other hand – although she feels that social services 'want to know more' – is quite happy with the fact that her social worker comes to check on how her money is being spent from time to time. 'It doesn't bother me, they're pretty good, they give me quite a bit.' Dorothy is in her fifties, has several years experience of employing people and is confident of running her own life. Malcolm, on the other hand, is in his early twenties and has not long left residential care. It may be, therefore, that his social worker does not share Malcolm's confidence that he can establish his own ways of doing things. Whereas non-disabled people in their early twenties are expected to be able to leave the parental home and organise their own lives, it may be that there is not a similar expectation of disabled people. However, it would also be fair to say that few young non-disabled people take on the responsibilities of an employer and that disabled young people therefore have not only to be more competent but also to prove their competence in order to achieve independence as young adults.

Wages or cash in hand?

Malcolm takes pride in his ability to sort out the wages for his workers. He calculates tax and national insurance, receiving administrative assistance from a volunteer on a local youth employment project. 'I'm training him on computers and he sorts my files out.' Ironically, this help which he needs to carry out his role as an employer cannot be paid for by ILF money as such assistance does not qualify as 'personal care'. When Mark started to employ helpers direct rather than using an agency, 'I was worried about the national insurance and tax but I mentioned it to this friend who is an accountant and he said don't worry he will be able to do everything for me ... so he is sorting all this out for me.'

Although a number of other people also either dealt with tax and national insurance themselves or got help with doing this, some others treated their workers as self-employed. This was particularly likely to be the case where personal assistants worked on a short-term basis and/or for only a few hours each week or were living in and only being paid a low wage. Sources of funding encourage this practice in that the ILF does not take account of deductions for tax or national insurance in the way that it calculates awards and social services departments also seemed reluctant to do so.

Inadequate financial resources for personal assistance often meant, therefore, that 'cash in hand' had to be offered in order to attract potential workers. Because many people specifically did not want to employ someone with qualifications or experience in this kind of work and wanted instead someone who was prepared to be very flexible, they were able to tap into what might be called an 'informal' labour market.

This means that the types of people interested in this kind of work either tended to be people who, as Patrick put it, 'wanted time out' for whatever reason – often young people in transition, sometimes from abroad – or those who wanted casual, part-time work because of child-care or other commitments, or because they were on unemployment benefit or income support and could not get a job at a wage which made it worth their while coming off benefits.

Maria's current personal assistant, for example, is a young Australian woman, travelling the world. She is committed to staying with Maria for a year during which time she works in a video shop at weekends in order to save money (as the amount that Maria can afford to pay her for working during the week does not give her much opportunity to save).

Vicky also employs mostly young women from overseas, mainly because they are prepared to be flexible and thus enable her to live the kind of life she chooses. 'I don't think they have so many pre-set ideas, they just come in fresh, I suppose working in another country, and being on a sort of holiday, travelling, you do feel far fresher and happier in a different environment than maybe you do in your own environment. Most of them stay six to nine months, maybe sometimes a year ... It's quite sad when they have to leave but it's also healthy because then someone starts who's quite fresh and it's a whole new experience.' Vicky says, 'There's no way I can employ them if they wish to tax them' but she also finds the whole idea of calculating tax and national insurance very intimidating. 'Originally, when this whole idea of independent living was introduced to me by [the local disability organisation] they very much wanted to do it the correct way so we all had to get involved with the local tax office and we were suddenly all meant to have the ability to be accountants. Just like that. And although they showed us what to do and how to do it, I just can't deal with the figures. It wasn't so much the figures it was knowing what columns to put which figures and knowing what's deducted. It was just all ... it was just a real hassle and I just didn't want to do it ... I would have been quite happy if somebody, you know for me to ... obviously for me to have the money and decide what I pay, but then for somebody else to do the books ... but I would want it to be a private accountant, nobody to do with social services, possibly [the local disability organisation].'

One of the reasons that Julie left her job was that her employer, having agreed to fund the cost of personal assistance while she was at work, wanted to formalise the payment which meant that her helpers would have to pay tax and national insurance. This created a problem because Julie only needed help for a few hours a week and believed that she wouldn't find the helpers unless it was cash in hand. 'I pay the people I employ cash in hand because for the hours I need them ... which isn't all the time ... nobody is going to come off the dole to work for that number of hours. And I don't pay them a bad wage, like, it's £3 cash in hand ... and if I paid them a proper wage it would be like £4.50 or something. I'd be quite happy to do that but for the hours I need them, it's just not worth them coming off the dole.'

Even Lauren, who can offer her personal assistants a full-time salaried position and whose funding takes account of the costs of being an employer, finds that she sometimes needs to employ people on a cash-in-hand basis to cover the extra four hours in the afternoon that she has in addition to the 12-hour shifts worked by her full-time helpers. Apart from one area where a personal assistance service run by a disability organisation was able to offer a swift response from workers known to its users, agencies are the only other source of finding workers for a few hours a week. Many people are not willing to use agencies, partly because they are expensive and partly because there is then limited control over the nature of the help provided. The dilemma is no different, however, from that faced by those non-disabled people who employ cleaners and child-minders, most of whom also work for cash in hand.

Making the relationship work

There were some indications that those people who paid for the cost of their personal assistance themselves had a different sort of relationship with their helpers compared with the relationship with workers sent by the local authority. As Robin said, 'Now I've been doing it for a while, I'm quite clear about being able to tell them what to do ... not order them about, you know, but I think it's a clearer relationship ... also it's my home and they treat it as such.' And William, who uses his attendance allowance to employ some-one at weekends – because he can't get his social services authority to provide help then – says, 'It can be really liberating ... I know who's coming and I know that he'll fit in with my plans ... well, it's not really a case of fitting in, he's paid to do it ... it's just so much less hassle.'

However, paying money to someone for the help they provide is not all there is to a relationship with a paid personal assistant. Some people consciously put a lot of effort into making the relationship with personal assistants as easy as possible. Dorothy has a number of helpers coming in to provide 24-hour assistance and is very aware that it only works if she gets on well with them. This involves being sensitive to their needs, 'You've got to treat people carefully and have a good relationship with them.' When she interviews people 'we reach an understanding that I want them to do things the way I like them done. I don't like to be domineered by anybody. Also it's my home and I have to have it run the way I want it run. I tell them all that at the interview.' However, her assertion of autonomy is done very sensitively: 'I feel that if someone wasn't doing things the way I want them to I would just have to tell them. But in a nice sort of way.' Moreover, she is reluctant to take herself off to her bedroom when she wants privacy as 'I suppose they might feel I was being a bit anti-social.' Instead, she says, 'I can do things while they're there. They can watch television and I would write my letters or make jewellery.'

Dorothy hopes that her helpers will stay with her for a reasonable period of time as she finds that changes can be very disruptive. Patrick, on the other hand, prefers his helpers to stay for only 6 months. 'I think I find somebody new a challenge. It stimulates me. I also think that, because they live in, after about six months you get to the stage where they're just going through the motions.' However, he says: 'It's not always like that. I did have one carer who lived here for a year and it was just brilliant. He was the sort of person who could take himself off and do his own thing. It's very important that he was able to create that space away from me for himself, that I didn't have to push him into it.'

Patrick says that he doesn't want to feel responsibility for his live-in helpers when they are off duty, 'I don't want to entertain them.' However, he is also aware that he does give a lot of support to helpers. This is inevitable because his main source of recruitment is an agency which finds work in Britain for Scandinavian young people. 'I give them emotional support to a point. I don't carry them. I establish this at the interview and sometimes I have to say 'it's not my problem'. It's usually OK. If they have problems or difficulties I direct them to other sources of help'.

Maria feels that she offers both emotional support to her helpers and 'generally the bonus of an interesting time because I do go out a lot'. When she interviews people she tries to assess whether a potential employee will be able to fit into her life in a way which allows for a harmonious coexistence. 'I always think it's such a difficult relationship. You start with someone whom you don't know at all and suddenly you're on a very intimate basis because of the nature of the work. For a start, you whip your clothes off very quickly. It never used to bother me before, when I was a dancer, because my body was quite nice. But that's always the first thing you feel you have to apologise for, the way things look these days. I don't think my body's very nice. Depending on who helps me, those personal things can be smoothed over with someone that I get on with. But if it's somebody who I don't feel very in tune with, it can be much worse, because I feel "damn it, I want to do this myself, but I've got to have somebody and so I've got to rely on you". This sounds awful, I sound a real bitch, but I suppose things become more irritating and frustrating because of that. If you don't get on with someone, the things they are doing for you are so personal – like inserting a tampon – that it can be very difficult. Sometimes I make a bad judgement about someone and other times I am forced to take on someone I'm not completely happy with, especially for weekend work. It's very difficult to tell whether you're really going to get on with someone at an interview. It's not until they start work that you can really get to know them. And they also find it difficult to know whether they are going to like working for me until they actually do it.'

The second time Maria was interviewed she had just taken on a new personal assistant after a period of uncertainty and fluctuations and she talked about the difference it made to her life to have someone who fitted in well. 'I've struck extremely lucky as far as [the new personal assistant] is concerned. She's a very thoughtful person to have around. It's great ... I feel I can àsk her to do things and she'll do them without any problems ... I realise during the weeks that I didn't have anybody here with me who knew my routine really well so that I didn't have to keep repeating everything and so it didn't take so long to do things ... my working life almost stopped. I just couldn't function. It would take so much longer to get up in the morning, it's hard to explain really but you just feel like you're in limbo waiting for some security. It's happened very quickly with her, she's very quick to pick up things. It isn't enough to have somebody there to do things, you need a rapport and an ease with being with someone. It doesn't always happen but when it does it's like breathing a sigh of relief. When I don't have somebody like that my work is getting my personal care sorted out, if I do have someone like that it just all happens in the background.'

Maria worries about whether her helpers get bored if, say, she has a day at home. 'At the interview, I ask them whether they've got any hobbies that they can do while we're at home because that helps.' She also feels responsible for whether they are enjoying themselves if, for example, she has friends round – 'I don't mind them being around when my friends come round as long as they can join in and I don't feel I have to bring them into the conversation. That kind of thing can be very wearing.' And being on her own, or with a lover, can become an uncomfortable issue. 'It's sometimes like having a gooseberry around. If they are not sensitive and remove themselves from the room the only private time I would have with [a lover] would be when I was in bed with them. Which isn't enough. I have always found it difficult to say to someone I want to be on my own.'

Balancing one's own needs and those of a paid helper can be extremely difficult, particularly for those people who need 24-hour assistance. These difficulties are to some extent an inevitable part of the need to have someone available for 24-hours a day. Lauren, who works full-time and also looks after her son and her mother, said, 'It's like having three quite responsible jobs – a senior position at work, managing four workers, which is more difficult than managing in a work setting, and caring.' She talked about how she deals with any problems which may come up with a personal assistant. 'There's a very fine line between being a friend and being a boss., I still retain the position that at the end of the day I am a boss and if I don't like what they're doing then they have to go. I have had a few occasions when someone has totally pissed me off and I have had to tell them. It is difficult though. I usually tend to tell them just before they go to bed because then they've got the whole night to sulk about it. It's very difficult because if you've got such a close relationship and you tell them off in the morning and they're doing things for you all day in a resentful way – even if they're not resentful they're obviously going to feel something so it's better for them to have all night to get over it. It's a terrible thing to say but I've sometimes had them in tears but it's all sorted out with a cigarette and a cuddle.'

When Ian first employed a personal assistant when he moved out of residential care he found it difficult to maintain an employer/employee relationship. 'She was with me for 18 months but it didn't really work. I think because she was very young and unfortunately it was the first time I had ever done any independent living and I tended to treat her very much almost like a surrogate daughter and it was a very great mistake. Because she wasn't particularly an honest girl and I was a stupid person at the time. Unfortunately she managed to con quite a lot of money and stuff out of me.'

The next person that Ian employed was older but she too wanted to borrow money from him. 'She does hassle a lot about money, she never seems to have any money to live by and occasionally she borrows some money from me but to be fair she always pays it back. But it does get to a stage where I'm forever listening about her financial problems which I find is a form of harassment, up to a point ... It's quite a mental responsibility because she leaves you with all this sort of thing, should I take some money and give it to her, you know, this kind of thing ... She's already borrowed one tenner this week from me and she's already going on and on about other things and I think quite honestly I am beginning to wonder whether she is thinking that I am an easy touch, which is the problem I had with the previous girl.'

However, by the time Ian was interviewed again things had settled down. 'I now know how to let all her waffle drift over me kind of thing ... We're friendly, but I try not to enter into her dialogue, or her monologue rather, it's best left, it's rather like having a heath fire, just let it burn out ... I did make a point that I wasn't a bank and that one of the points that the other girl left on was that she'd kept on at me about money and I think the actual sort of point was taken. She does still occasionally borrow £5 for petrol but she always pays me back. I think it does work rather nicely now.' One of the reasons that he had persevered with this helper was that the physical help that she had given him was, as he put it, 'superb', and this was an important skill which he wanted to hang on to.

Employing people can be difficult, particularly when the funding of personal assistance does not take into account all the costs involved. Those who received help from other disabled people and from disability organisations valued both peer support and practical advice. People who employed personal assistants found that over the years they built up the skills necessary to assess who would make a suitable personal assistant for them, and also developed the confidence to deal with any problems in the relationship.

Those people who had the money to pay for personal assistance were generally able to have the kind of control over their lives which was not possible for those solely reliant on either services or on family and friends. This kind of control was important, not only for those who lived on their own, but also for those people living with partners, parents and/or children.

Part III
Policy Implications: Prospects for the Future

9

Community care or independent living?

The people whose experiences are explored in Part II confront daily the issues raised by the development of community care policies. We conclude this book by looking at how far the 1990/93 community care reforms are likely to contribute to the disability movement's goal of independent living.

Important progress

During the 1980s, the disability movement at its international, national and local levels of organisation started to bring about important changes in general attitudes towards impairment and in the status of disabled people. While there is a long way to go at least disability is now on the political agenda as a civil rights issue.

Disabled people themselves are increasingly asserting the changes they need to secure their human and civil rights. The challenges thrown out by the disability movement are reflected in the way that some individuals approach their relationships with non-disabled people as well as the way that they approach organisations which have the resources necessary to achieve independent living. Patrick, for example, gained important information and confirmation of his right to leave residential care from his contact with another disabled man who was involved in the independent living movement. This helped to give him a strong sense that he was making a legitimate demand on his local authority housing department. Jackie's identification of what she calls 'able-bodied behaviour' is one example of the developments in disabled people's own consciousness and expectations in the context of personal relationships. Valuing herself as a disabled woman enables Jackie to resist 'things that are exclusive of me or taking over. They're the two sins really aren't they? Taking you over and pushing you out.'

The disability movement's articulation of the medical and social models of disability and the insistence that it is attitudes and environments which disable people have started to influence even the government's attitude. In the 1992 General Election campaign Nicholas Scott, Conservative Minister for Disabled People, told the Greater Manchester Coalition of Disabled People:

> The Government's principal aims which guide and inform policies affecting disabled people are to enable disabled people to maximise their individual potential, to live independently where possible, to have employment opportunities and to enjoy their leisure time ... Increasingly, disabled people will demand control over their own lives. Government, local and national, as well as the voluntary and charitable sectors, will need to adjust to this new, demanding, but exciting situation.
>
> (*GMCDP Information Sheet*, vol. 2, no. 1, 27 March 1992)

A recognition of disabled people's right to control over their own lives is reflected in some of the rhetoric associated with community care policies. The Foreword to the White Paper *Caring for People* opens with the statement, 'Helping people to lead, as far as possible, full and independent lives is at the heart of the Government's approach to community care.' And the White Paper's first paragraph states, 'The Government is firmly committed to a policy of community care which enables ... people to achieve their full potential.'

When the Social Services Inspectorate produced its guide for local authorities on developing assessment procedures, the first two principles identified concerned enabling people to 'live a full life in the community' and to 'be in charge of their own lives and make their own decisions including decisions to take risks' (Social Services Inspectorate, 1991a, p. 6.)

At a local level, the rhetoric of community care uses similar terms. A number of Community Care Plans include statements about a commitment to enabling people to live independent lives. This type of statement, made at local and national level, by both politicians and professionals, is compatible with the independent living movement's assertion that disability is a civil rights issue, and that both central and local government policy should be concerned with removing the barriers to disabled people's full participation in society.

However, this compatibility is actually a superficial one. The aim of independent living, of full and equal participation in society, is held back by an ideology which does not recognise the civil rights of disabled people but instead considers them to be dependent people and in need of care.

The ideology of caring

It is important to reiterate clearly what is meant by the terms 'care' and 'caring', building on the analysis presented in Chapter 3. In the context of the political, professional and academic debates on community care, 'care' – whether it refers to people giving paid or unpaid help – does not mean to 'care about' someone, in the sense of loving them. Rather it means to 'care for' someone, in the sense of taking responsibility for them, taking charge of them. As Elizabeth put it so succinctly when describing the nature of the help she receives from the Family Aides employed by her social services department, 'They want to give help in a ... custodial sense rather than facilitate ... When you're being custodial you're ... well, you're dictating aren't you, more or less, you're smothering a person's sense of independence.'

The custodial nature of the role of carers as paid workers (which has traditionally been particularly strong within residential/institutional provision and has been carried over into domiciliary services) has heavily influenced the way that family members have become identified as carers. Those who have a personal relationship with a disabled person and who provide them with some form of help have been constructed as 'informal carers'. The word 'informal' is used to distinguish them from carers who are paid to help as a job but the common definition of 'carer' is much more heavily associated with the 'taking charge of' definition of care than it is with the 'caring about' definition.

The custodial nature of caring is further buttressed by the way that social and economic inequalities resulting from impairment influence disabled people's interaction with others. Disabled people often find it difficult to resist being 'taken charge of' by family members, or by paid carers. Rosemary's experience, for example, of being protected by her mother, and discouraged for many years from even going out of the house, was very different from that of her non-disabled sister whose transition to adulthood was marked, unlike Rosemary's, by getting a job, getting married and leaving home.

The term 'care', applied as it is to both paid workers and to family members to mean taking charge of someone, is based on the notion of 'dependent people'. Impairment is assumed to reduce the ability of disabled people to look after themselves and this is why they are called 'dependent people' – they are assumed to depend on others to take responsibility for their well-being.

When applied to people with physical impairments, the assumption of dependency is seen as having both physical and/or intellectual causes. In a physical sense, some types of impairment mean that someone cannot do practical things for themselves, such as getting in and out of bed. On the intellectual or emotional level, people with physical impairments are often seen as unable to make decisions that would be in their own best interests.

We have seen, however, that the independent living movement strongly challenges the assumption that physical inability to perform daily living tasks inevitably creates dependency. The experiences explored in Part II of this book illustrate how it is the *way* that physical impairment is responded to which creates dependency rather than the impairment itself. Kavita, for example, described how she is made dependent by inappropriate housing and a reliance on her sister and mother for help. Yet Maria, who has a higher level of physical impairment than Kavita, says that employing personal assistants enables her to 'lead the kind of life that I want to'.

But, say critics of the independent living movement, it is only certain kinds of people who can assert control over their lives. Many people are not mentally capable of doing so, or do not wish to do so, and some people are a danger to themselves and others unless someone takes responsibility for them. The problem here is that it is the perspectives and values of non-disabled people generally, and health and social services professionals in particular, which dominate judgements about disabled people in respect of capability, risks, acceptable behaviour and desirable outcomes.

While it may be that some people with physical impairments are not able, or do not wish, to take over responsibility for their personal assistance requirements, we cannot trust such an assessment within the current community care context because the reaction to and experience of impairment is so much dominated by the assumption that physical impairment inevitably creates dependency. The social context of impairment does not enable disabled children to make the transition to independent adulthood or adults who acquire an impairment to retain their independence and autonomy. As Richard Wood says:

> So strong is [the] medical model of disability that many disabled people have also come to believe that they must let others manage their lives since they are not competent to do so themselves. Thus, disabled people's lives are often dominated by professionals and services which de-skill us and turn us into passive recipients of care (Wood, 1991, p. 200).

Critics of the disability movement also argue that the goals of independent living are not applicable to the majority of disabled people who are old and/or experience poor health. Proponents of independent living are accused of addressing only the concerns of young, fit, predominantly male, wheelchair users. Yet, if we accept the basic premise of the independent living movement – namely that all human life has value – then it is difficult to deny that the human and civil rights that younger, fitter, more articulate disabled people are claiming for themselves should also be accorded to those who are older and/or less articulate.

We have seen from this study how important control over personal assistance is to people like Bob and Robin whose impairments are associated with being ill. As Robin says, 'I don't think people understand that when you're ill it's even more important to have control over the help you get, when you get it and how they ... how someone does things.' Feminists have made the case over the past twenty years of how important it is for women to have control over their bodies, both in reproductive terms and in the context of experiences such as cancer. It is no different for those men and women who are defined as dependent because of old age and/or impairment.

To argue that, because many people with physical impairments are currently unable to assert control over their lives, the goals of independent living are not applicable to them, is to adopt the same position as those who argued in the last century that working-class people should not have the vote because they could not read or write.

Community care policies should be measured against the goal of furthering disabled people's human and civil rights, rather than starting from the position that some people need 'taking charge of', i.e. need care. We particularly need to challenge assumptions that are made about relationships between disabled people and their families. The human and civil rights of disabled people, like those of women, are closely bound up with the nature of their personal relationships. The feminist challenge to women's position in society included a challenge to the assumption that men have the right to 'take charge of' women's lives. A similar challenge must be mounted to the nature of relationships where one party has a physical or sensory impairment (or indeed an intellectual impairment or is old). Caring *about* someone does not bestow the right to make choices for them, to curtail their autonomy, just because they have a physical impairment, any more than marriage confers the right on men to control women. Neither does the state, in the form of care managers, care workers, have the right to take charge of a disabled person's life, any more than the state has the right to take charge of a woman's fertility.

This research has firmly established that, where someone does not have control over the help which they need, their human and their civil rights suffer. For some this means being confined more or less to where they live (whether this is their own home or in residential care), unable to enter into personal relationships, seek employment or engage in leisure activities. For others, the level and type of help they receive not merely creates a low quality of life but can damage their health.

For some people, the isolation and powerlessness associated with the custodial nature of caring results in serious abuse. The experiences of physical and sexual abuse which were revealed during some of the interviews all took place in a context where a disabled person was being 'cared for', whether by a paid carer, a partner or family member. There is very little recognition of disabled people's experience of abuse. Indeed the use of words like 'carers' and 'caring' contribute to a refusal to confront the reality of being made dependent, of being made powerless.

Policy-makers, professionals and service deliverers who are committed to disabled people's rights to be equal citizens are continually struggling against the ideology of caring which dominates community care policies, often not recognising its constraints. The changes brought in by the 1990 legislation have at their heart the concept of dependent people and a reliance on informal carers. Yet the rhetoric accompanying the changes, and the genuine commitment of some policy-makers and professionals, often seems to be aimed at progressing the civil rights of disabled people. Indeed, at times, it seems as if two philosophies are struggling for coexistence within community care policy.

We will now look at three particular ways in which people receive personal assistance – from family and friends, local authority home care services and by paying for help. The experiences of these three forms of help which were explored in Part II all have implications for the implementation of community care policies.

Informal care and dependency

The experiences set out in Part II of this book clearly illustrate the way that a reliance on assistance solely provided by family and friends is incompatible with the philosophy of independent living. Those people who have significant personal assistance requirements and who have been able to participate fully in society and in personal relationships, have done so *because* they have not had to rely solely on family and friends for the help they need. Lauren, for example, who needs assistance with all daily living tasks, can only work, bring up her son and, now, look after her mother, because she employs people to do all the things with which she needs help.

Reliance on a family member creates significant restraints on the autonomy of both the disabled person and the person providing the help. Lauren's personal assistants are doing a job when they enable her to go to work and run her home; they work 12-hour shifts and hand over to another worker at the end of each shift. A family member could only provide the same type of assistance by totally sublimating their own lives and needs to that of the person for whom they are providing assistance, and such a situation would, in the process, change beyond recognition the personal relationship.

It is not surprising therefore that those who rely on family or friends are unlikely to be able to go out to work and indeed any activity outside the home may be significantly curtailed because there is a limit to the assistance which such a helper can provide. Ibrahim's reliance on his father, for example, means that his basic physical needs are more or less met, but he is mostly confined to his home. Robin's dependence on his mother for assistance meant that he had to give up his job following his injury and he could not pursue an independent social life.

This is not to deny that many people with personal assistance requirements would – even when alternative help is available – *choose* to have some of those needs met within a personal relationship. Giving, and receiving, personal assistance can be an expression of love, as both Bob and Moira found, and therefore an important part of a relationship. Moreover, as Gillian Parker points out:

> the provision of personal support services from outside [a relationship] is likely both to threaten certain sorts of relationships, particularly established marriages, and to run counter to what some disabled people within those relationships want (Parker, 1992, p. 254).

As Catherine's experience highlighted, there are also relationships where the non-disabled partner wishes to provide all or most of the help whereas the disabled person appreciates the independence that outside help can bring.

It is also important to recognise that there is not always a neat division within households between those who need help with daily living tasks, and are 'dependent', and those who give help, and are 'carers'. Many disabled people, such as those whose lives are explored in Chapter 6, experience relationships with partners, children, parents where they give physical and/or emotional support. Indeed, it must be stressed that receiving help from those with whom a disabled person has a personal relationship does not turn them into carers – nor the disabled person into a dependent. In Chapter 3 we discussed the fact that most people classified as carers by both community care policy and by pressure group politics do not see themselves as such. It can also be argued that few disabled people see themselves as having a carer. None of those interviewed for this book who received help from family members referred to those family members as carers. Instead they talked about 'my mother', 'my husband', 'my wife', 'my partner'. They talked about their relationships not about their carers.

Research on informal carers has recognised that the nature of the relationship between the two parties involved is very important in determining the experience of providing assistance. The experiences explored in this research project illustrate how important it is for those receiving help from a partner or other family member. Robin, for example, does not see his wife as his carer. Neither does he see himself as being cared for or dependent. Instead, he sees himself as Laura's husband and both the practicalities and emotional consequences of the assistance he needs are worked out in the context of their relationship. For him it is an equal and reciprocal relationship, unlike that which he experienced with his mother. The contrast in his two experiences of receiving assistance within a personal relationship illustrates how the nature of the relationship determines the experience of giving and receiving assistance.

However, the social construction of informal carers, and in particular the assumption that caring is about taking charge of someone, diminishes relationships. Rather than assuming that the presence of a non-disabled family member creates a relationship of carer and cared-for, it is the relationship between partners, parent and child, siblings, etc. which should be recognised. Some relationships can sustain the giving of personal assistance, some cannot. Some people can facilitate independence for their partner, parent or child, some cannot. Some relationships are abusive and exploitative, some are liberating. To categorise people as carers and dependents is to gloss over all of this.

Independent living is not only an issue for those who live on their own, or for those who are physically fit. A very damaging stereotype has been constructed of a young, single, wheelchair user for whom paid personal assistance is an issue because s/he has no family on which to depend. In contrast, it is assumed that those who live with a partner, parents or children want to/should be looked after by family members and the focus is therefore on supporting informal carers. Yet a number of people interviewed for this study who were living in family households identified the importance of help being provided by those who were paid to give it. Such help was vital not only to prevent them being totally dependent on family members and enabling them to make independent choices, but also to enable people to participate in family relationships on an equal basis. Jackie, for example, talked about the kind of help she needed to enable her both to contribute to household tasks and to play her role as a parent. All this was crucial to maintaining her relationship: 'If there's quite a good balance in my life in terms of getting support and being able to do things in different ways and in different environments and stuff then it's really lovely to have Ros doing things for me because it's part of a loving relationship. But when it goes out of balance and it seems to be only Ros it's absolutely dreadful and you lose sight of the fact that we're lovers and that we're individuals and that we do actually love each other, because there's no space for it left.'

From the perspective of the independent living movement, community care policies are fatally flawed by the central importance which is given to the role of informal carers. The social construction of informal carers undermines relationships, creates dependency and denies autonomy. This process is experienced both by those constructed as carers and by those constructed as dependent people.

Local authority home care services

During the second half of the 1980s, most social services authorities started to grapple with the issue of whether their home help service could, as a Social Services Inspectorate (SSI) report put it, 'be the backbone of a support service offering practical and personal care for people who under previous policies would have been cared for in institutions' or whether 'different kinds of domiciliary care and support services [are] required for such policies to be fulfilled?' (Social Services Inspectorate, 1987, p. 2). Traditionally, home helps did housework and shopping and the majority of users of the service did not receive significant help with personal care tasks. People who needed such help either relied on informal carers or entered residential care, although a few younger disabled people managed to get their social services department to respond to their personal assistance needs through direct or indirect payments, or through volunteer schemes such as that run by Community Service Volunteers. Such response was often on an *ad hoc* basis and not part of a formal policy of planning for the needs of younger disabled people.

During the 1980s, the development of policies on domiciliary services, at both central and local government level, was almost totally dominated by addressing the needs of old people, and in particular, very old people. The 1987 SSI report pointed out:

If increasing numbers of very elderly people are to be enabled to continue living in their own homes, or in sheltered housing, rather than having to move into residential care, *either* a higher volume of domiciliary services will be necessary, *or* the currently available resources will have to be more specifically targeted on those in most need, and those for whom most can be achieved. The nature of the services provided will also have to change significantly (SSI, 1987, p. 26, emphasis in original).

Any increase in resources available to local authorities for expenditure on domiciliary services during the later 1980s was generally taken up by the increasing number of people over the age of 75. There was therefore little potential to expand existing home help services in order *also* to provide more help with personal care. Thus the shift from home help (cleaning and shopping) to home care (help with personal care, taking of medicines, etc.) and accompanying 'substantial changes in *who* gets services, *what kinds* of support they receive, and *when* they receive it' (SSI, 1987, p. 26, emphasis in original.)

Most local authority home help services have been renamed home care services and are targeted at those most at risk of entering residential care, primarily those identified as 'frail elderly people'. The way that the service is delivered, however, creates a number of conflicts between the principles of independent living and the implementation of community care policies.

A reduction in choice

As a result of the change in the nature of domiciliary services a number of people interviewed for this study found that they could no longer get help with housework. Maeve complained that when her home help went on long-term sick leave she was never replaced, Tricia's home-help hours were reduced and Marcia was told that home helps no longer did housework.

These are experiences which were also found amongst those surveyed by RADAR and Arthritis Care in 1990/91 (RADAR and Arthritis Care, 1991). Their survey highlighted the way that many local authorities had adopted a formal policy of reducing the amount of help with housework, pointing out that this was probably in contravention of statutory duties. 'Practical assistance in the home', provided under Section 2 of the Chronically Sick and Disabled Persons Act, should not be withdrawn or reduced in the absence of a diminution of need, according to legal advice given by the Department of Health and Social Security in 1975 (RADAR and Arthritis Care, 1991, p. 1). Yet some local authorities, in order to reallocate resources to those whose personal assistance needs placed them at risk of entering residential care, instructed home help organisers to reduce the amount of help given with housework and to provide no relief cover when home helps went on holiday or were off sick.

The rationing of local authority domiciliary services has created a situation where a need for help with housework is generally given little priority. As the RADAR/Arthritis Care report said:

> There appears to be a genuine lack of understanding in social services departments about how important a clean home is to people who, in many cases, have to spend the majority of their lives inside their homes. Apart from their distress in living in what they see as unhygienic surroundings they also feel painfully humiliated at having to sit and look at what they see as degradation and by being told that housework is not important (RADAR, 1991, p. 1).

It is clear from the experiences of those interviewed for this study that disabled people's ability to choose how their needs for assistance are met is significantly undermined by a reliance on home care services. For example, some people prefer personal care tasks to be carried out by a family member, and would welcome help with housework to reduce the amount of work that they have to ask of those with whom they live. Such a choice is often not possible under the priorities set by home care services and some people interviewed for this research project found that if help with such tasks was given by a family member or by a paid personal assistant, then they did not qualify for any help with housework.

The general experience of those interviewed who relied on home care services for help with daily living tasks was that services were often not flexible enough to enable them to make the most elementary choices such as when to get up and when to go to bed – or even when to go to the toilet.

Even when a service is agreed, this does not always mean that people get the tasks done which they want doing in the way that they want. Elizabeth could not get the Family Aides to do her hair in the way she wanted, or to cook the particular food she wanted. This type of experience is in contrast to the personal assistance service run by a disability organisation where users were allocated a certain number of hours of assistance but were free to use the help provided in whatever way they chose. This is what control over personal assistance requirements is all about.

Undermining relationships

The way that local authority services are delivered generally does not recognise people's role within their household. For example, when Jackie temporarily needed help after a fall, she wanted help with the tasks that she normally contributed to her household – cooking, doing the washing, and other domestic tasks. All that was on offer, however, was help with personal-care tasks such as getting up and dressed. Robin argued that he wanted someone to do the things that he would otherwise have done, such as 'putting together a self-assembly wardrobe, sticking the leg back on a chair – I don't see why my wife should go out to work, come home to do the housework, look after me *and* do all those other things that I would have done if I hadn't had my accident.' Again all that was on offer from his local authority was help with personal care tasks.

Women in particular – given expectations of their role within the family – are likely to want help with carrying out all the tasks associated with running a home and bringing up children. Moira said, 'There's no way I could rely on home care ... they wouldn't treat me like a mother, with, you know, like ... responsibilities for my child.' Instead, she would be treated solely as someone in need of personal care, rather than as a carer herself who needed practical help in order to be a parent.

Elizabeth said that her Family Aides thought that they should not help her with, for example, cooking or eating, if she had friends or members of her family round 'You can't have human relationships because they're making me dependent', echoing a number of people who felt that their ability to maintain family relationships and friendships was undermined by an assumption that if family or friends were present this then diminished their priority for services.

Fitting the client to the criteria

Those who want or need to use their local authority's home care services find themselves having to fit their requirements into the service's criteria and these can sometimes bear little relationship to their own assessment of the situation. William, for example, had to argue that help with washing his clothes was related to incontinence. In his view, he needed help because he couldn't get the clothes into and out of the washing machine himself; from the home care service's point of view he had to fit into a priority category based on medical/hygiene needs.

Elizabeth's access to the Meals-on-Wheels service was threatened when she started to work part-time and wanted a meal delivered to her workplace (which was across the road from her home). The Meals-on-Wheels service operated on the assumption that its clients were 'housebound', whereas Elizabeth needed the service because the way her arms shake makes cooking difficult, dangerous and tiring. A number of people in this study found, like William and Elizabeth, that assessments and prioritising for services tend to focus on dependency, instead of identifying what is necessary for independence.

Unequal treatment

The 1987 SSI report found variations within local authority areas of demand and take-up of home care services. In this current research project, even though many people experienced their home care service as operating fairly rigid eligibility criteria which it was often difficult to meet, there were, within each of the four areas in which the interviewees lived, very significant differences in the likelihood of their receiving a service and in the level of service delivered. One example is the contrasting experience of Maeve and Marcia who both have similar levels of impairment (with the same physical cause). Maeve receives less informal care than Marcia yet, at the time of interview, she had been refused help from the home care service whereas Marcia had just been allocated a service. The only difference in their situations which could account for this was that Marcia had closer links with disability organisations and was able to rely on one worker in particular to help her to get the service she needed, whereas Maeve was completely isolated.

Such experiences highlight the importance of implementing Section 1 of the 1986 Disabled Persons Act which would give someone like Maeve the right to an advocacy service.

Institutionalisation within the community

Another key feature of local authority domiciliary services is their assumption that users of the service are confined, more or less, to their own home. This is very much related to the fact that the major users of home care services are very old people – the 1987 SSI report found that 88 per cent of home care service users were 'elderly, with over two-thirds aged 75 and over'. In a sense local authority home carers are carrying out a service which otherwise would have been carried out in a residential establishment. A number of people found that going out of their home – whether to work or for leisure activities – did not fit in with the assumptions of the service and indeed sometimes a domiciliary service was withdrawn if they started work or college. As Valerie said: 'I think the community care philosophy doesn't understand what independent living is ... They seem to think that community care is about someone being cosy and comfortable, being kept clean. To me that's a step back into the situation of residential care – living in the contained environment of your own home. If you don't broaden it out it isn't independent living.'

Some people appreciate the way that home care services can take over the responsibility for ensuring that personal assistance is provided and would not want to recruit and employ their own helpers. People like Jackie particularly appreciate her local authority's equal opportunities policies which, she says, means that she knows that a home care worker will not discriminate against her as a lesbian. However, the lack of control over the type of help which is given means that people who have particular requirements arising from their cultural needs (such as some of the Asian and Afro-Caribbean respondents in this study) often find that these requirements are not met.

The general context in which home care services are delivered, and the principles on which they operate, are in conflict with the concept of independent living. Disabled people who have to rely solely on local authority domiciliary services are at risk of being confined within their own homes and of their personal relationships being undermined by the failure to recognise their role within their household. Moreover, the shift from home help to home care has, for many people, resulted in contraventions of their rights under the 1970 Chronically Sick and Disabled Persons Act.

Paying for assistance

The experiences of those people who received cash to pay for the assistance that they need illustrates the potential for achieving independent living. Rather than being cared for, those who employ personal assistants are paying for tasks to be done which enable them to assert control over their lives. The purchase of assistance is clearly a means to an end. In contrast, the delivery of home care services is often seen as an end in itself. The Independent Living Fund concluded from its own research on recipients of ILF grants that:

> The choice and control they valued so highly could not in their experience be provided by statutory authorities. It is not simply a matter of resource levels, though these are very significant. As important are the qualities that any large-scale service-providing organisation would find hard to deliver: choice of care assistant, flexibility, consistency, control of times and tasks, etc. (Kestenbaum, 1992, p. 77).

Most people who employed personal assistants, when asked what the term independent living meant to them, referred first to the ability to choose how and when to do the very basic activities of getting up, going to bed, eating, drinking, going to the toilet. However, they then went on to talk about how this meant that they could engage in employment or leisure activities and participate in personal and social relationships. For Vicky, control over when she goes to bed meant she could stay up until 3 in the morning preparing for a course she was doing; for Maria paying someone to help her with daily living tasks means that her physical needs do not get in the way of relationships with family and friends; and for Jack control over personal assistance means, as he put it 'I'm a husband, a father and a breadwinner.'

Independent living is about both human and civil rights. If disabled people do not have control over the very basic activities of daily living then they cannot hope even to begin to participate in society on an equal basis. Independent living also has major equal opportunities implications. Control over personal assistance is the only way to meet the requirements which arise in specific contexts because of factors associated with gender, race and sexuality. It certainly seems the most effective way of fulfilling one of the principles laid down in the SSI's guidance on assessment procedures, namely, that SSDs should enable people to 'have their cultural, ethnic, religious, sexual and emotional needs recognised and respected' (Social Services Inspectorate, 1991a, p. 6).

Before going on to look at some of the issues raised by the experience of paying for personal assistance in more detail it is, however, important to point out that while control over personal assistance is a necessary part of independent living, it is not usually sufficient. As the Audit Commission points out:

> Other community aspects besides social services are also important to users and carers [*sic*]. For example, is public transport accessible to physically disabled people? Can they use pavement crossings and pedestrian areas? Can they open doors to shopping precincts? Can people in wheelchairs gain access to shops and other public buildings? Do libraries provide material for those who are sensorily impaired? Is adult education available to people with mental and physical disabilities and is there access to appropriate housing or adaptations for all user groups? (Audit Commission, 1992, p. 28).

Social services authorities, as the lead agency on community care, will need to address these issues if the principle of independent living is to be incorporated wholeheartedly into their approach.

Are disabled people capable of managing the purchase of personal assistance?

One of the objections raised by various government ministers to the possibility of legalising direct payments was that, as Chancellor of the Exchequer, Norman Lamont, put it, 'many disabled people might have difficulty keeping records [required by SSDs for monitoring purposes] or might not want direct payments at all' (letter from Norman Lamont, dated 9 September 1992). The independent living movement's response to this is, first, that no one is saying that people should be forced to employ their own personal assistants, although many more wish to do so than the government initially thought to judge from the difference between the projected and the actual applications to the ILF. Second, the independent living movement points out that assumptions about disabled people's (in)capabilities are part of the prejudice and disadvantages which they currently experience. As Philip Mason writes:

The direct payment issue is a prime example of the sort of thing that will astound future generations. It will amaze people to think that there was a time when disabled people were thought unable or untrustworthy to receive, without hestitation, the finance that they need for the purchase and organisation of their own assistance (*Personal Assistance Users Newsletter*, April 1991, p. 3).

Few people today would argue that disabled people are incapable of purchasing the type of car best suited to their requirements and yet this was an argument which delayed the replacement of the three-wheeler 'invalid car' by a cash benefit in the form of the mobility allowance.

The Independent Living Fund itself has carried out research on those to whom it makes payments and concluded:

The findings from this research challenge the assumption that disabled people, even those with very severe disabilities, are incapable of exercising effective choice and control over their own care arrangements. It also shows that independent living is a relevant and important concept not only for the *young* disabled, but also for older people with many different kinds of disability. The experience of ILF clients detailed in this report shows how, with enough money to have care assistance under their own control or that of a chosen advocate, a wide range of severely disabled people can improve the quality of their lives as well as stay out of residential care (Kestenbaum, 1992, p. 78).

All this is not to deny, however, that there are often barriers created to independent living even when people receive the money to pay for personal assistance. Some of these barriers relate to the way the different systems of paying money operate, and some to the more general disadvantages experienced by disabled people.

Using Agencies

Some people undoubtedly appreciated and wanted help from social services professionals in using money to pay for assistance and in this kind of situation it is quite likely that the social services professional will turn to a private or voluntary agency service to supply personal assistance. Some disabled people also find it easier to use agencies rather than directly employ people themselves. The problem with both these situations is that possibilities are opened up for other people's priorities and expectations to dominate the way that assistance is provided rather than the priorities and expectations of the disabled person themselves. This was certainly true for Audrey who was confined to her home, and left alone for much of the day as a result of someone else determining what her personal assistance needs were.

It is interesting that, in this study, those who had real control over employing personal assistants all preferred to recruit people with little or no qualifications or experience of the work involved. People often found that personal assistants who had done this work before – particularly those who had worked in residential establishments – had set ideas about how things should be done, whereas each disabled employer has very particular needs and preferences. An inevitable disadvantage of using agency staff is that many of them will have previously worked (and some of them will be concurrently working) in residential establishments.

Using an agency can have distinct advantages, however, particularly in the event of a worker being off sick or on holiday when it will be the agency's responsibility rather than the user's task to arrange cover. Some people also feel that using a reputable agency will give them some protection from abuse and theft. That this is not necessarily the case was demonstrated by the murder of Cathy O'Neill – a woman who used personal assistance services – in 1991 by a worker employed by one of the better known London agencies.

The community care reforms envisage an increase in private agencies providing domiciliary services and it may well be that some disabled people who have control over their own personal assistance budgets will continue to choose to use agencies. Indeed, it is likely that social services professionals will encourage them to do so. In this situation it is very important that social services authorities do everything they can to ensure that agencies behave in a way which respects rather than undermines the autonomy of those who use their services.

It is unfortunate that there is, as yet, no obligation for private and voluntary domiciliary agencies to be registered with the local authority or requirement for them to be inspected (as there is with private and voluntary residential homes). Even before Cathy O'Neill's murder there was concern within the disability movement:

as to how to safeguard the interests of disabled people during a time when a whole new [domiciliary services] industry is burgeoning into fruition as the new community care legislation, with its endorsement of the independent sector, begins to take hold (*Personal Assistance Users Newsletter,* October 1992).

In response to this concern Hammersmith and Fulham Action on Disability drew up the following recommendations to promote quality of domiciliary services:

• Compulsory statutory registration of all private care agencies.
• Inspection to be carried out locally but under the auspices of the Social Services Inspectorate.
• Guidelines should include a check-list for registration, business plan specifications, their commitment to the involvement of users and personal assistants, quality assurance criteria and complaints procedures.
• Guidance should also be given on selection and recruitment procedures of personal assistants, training (which should include disability equality training) and supervision of personnel.

It is also important that care managers carefully weigh up the cost-effectiveness of using agencies before entering into such arrangements on behalf of personal assistance users. Such provision is usually the most costly, on an hourly basis, and the evidence from this study indicates that there are less expensive ways of purchasing personal assistance, ways which may, moreover, offer a higher quality of life for the user of personal assistance. Calculated on an hourly basis, it is almost always cheaper to employ someone direct than to use an agency and, in particular, those disabled people who employed personal assistants on weekly, rather than hourly, wages were able to purchase a greater quantity of more flexible personal assistance.

Indirect costs

The failure of direct payment systems (whether through social services departments or the ILF) to take account of the indirect costs of personal assistance poses unnecessary difficulties for those employing personal assistants. First, it means that costs such as extra expenditure on food, entertainment, transport, and even, sometimes, the employer's national insurance contribution have to come out of other income. Second, it tends to push users of personal assistants into bad employment practices, such as giving cash-in-hand and failing to take out employer's liability insurance. While this is not the only pressure to employing on a cash-in-hand basis – and such terms obviously suit some personal assistants very well – this practice is unlikely to be in the long-term interests of either users or personal assistants.

The ILF's failure to take account of indirect costs is clearly associated with its development of rationing mechanisms as the demands on its budget outstripped the increases agreed by the government. In the early days of the ILF's operation, when it was assumed that the budget would be sufficient to meet the needs of the few hundred people thought to be eligible, the principle which operated was that the ILF reimbursed the actual costs incurred of purchasing personal assistance. As it became clear that thousands of disabled people not only qualified for help from the ILF but very much wanted to purchase personal assistance, restrictions started to be placed, both on eligibility and on the way the grants were calculated.

Instead of reimbursing actual costs incurred, the ILF adopted a standard format for calculating grants awarded based on notional hourly rates paid for amount of assistance purchased. Not only did such hourly rates fail to relate to actual hourly rates paid but they also failed to take into account other costs such as VAT on agency bills and employers' national insurance contribution to wages bills. By 1992, the ILF's position was that it was only making a *contribution* to the costs of personal assistance – local authorities being expected to make up the difference. In reality, of course, as the ILF's Treasurer told the Hampshire Coalition of Disabled People:

> I am aware that in some cases our rules must mean that you can pay for fewer hours of care than are really needed, but coming back to the original reason, we do not have a bottomless purse and we have to try to make what we have go round in as fair a way as we can manage without involving tremendous administrative costs (*Personal Assistance Users' Newsletter*, December 1991, p. 7).

The need to ration scarce resources had, as he recognised, created a situation where people who had personal assistance requirements were not able to have those requirements fully met. Any system of funding personal assistance requirements which is not based on a system of rights, such as those enshrined in social security legislation, is likely to come up against similar needs to ration resources and will undoubtedly develop similar strategies which will lead to the under-resourcing of personal assistance.

Means-testing

If direct payment systems use a means test as a test of eligibility then disabled people's civil rights will be significantly undermined. A household means test will inhibit someone's right to live with a partner or family. One man interviewed for this study felt that he had to hide from his social services department the fact that his partner had moved in with him because his (in)direct payment was means-tested. They had discussed getting married but felt that this would be too risky. The prospect of this situation acting as a restriction on their decision whether or not to have a child was obviously causing some friction between them.

The Independent Living Fund has always operated a means test – and so will its successor body – but, in the early days, it was still possible for someone in work to receive a grant. Since August 1992, however, only those actually in receipt of Income Support can qualify for an ILF award. This not only creates a poverty trap – in that it is not in the interests of the recipient of an ILF award to seek employment – but it takes away people's right to seek employment.

If a direct payment system is truly to further disabled people's human and civil rights then it needs to be based on a principle of creating a 'level playing field'. The costs of personal assistance are only incurred because of physical impairment. Therefore people with personal assistance requirements can only begin to participate in society on an equal basis if they do not themselves have to pay the costs from whatever they may be able to earn.

Are direct payment systems cost-effective?

There is evidence that enabling people to employ their own personal assistants is a more cost-effective way of meeting personal assistance needs than using local authority home care services. Evaluation of the Personal Assistance Advisor post at Greenwich Association of Disabled People found that, even when allowing for the cost of the support and advice given by the Personal Assistance Advisor, employing personal assistants was cheaper than relying on health and social services. Indeed this was a point recognised by Conservative Minister Nicholas Scott in his Foreword to the report when he wrote,

> This report on Personal Assistance Schemes in Greenwich shows that as well as being cost effective, such schemes offer disabled people a greater degree of independence when compared with traditional forms of provision (Oliver and Zarb, 1992).

However, the evidence from this study also shows that there are wide variations in the cost of direct payments systems and that people may not always be getting the best value for their money. It is not possible to make accurate comparisions in real costs of the different personal assistance arrangements explored in Chapter 8 because hidden costs are rarely accounted for in the amount of cash received from the SSD and/or the ILF to pay for assistance. It is clear, however, that a reliance on agency staff can mean paying a relatively large sum of money for a service which is quite restrictive, as was discussed above.

When direct and indirect payments are made by SSDs this is rarely as a result of a formal policy but is often a response to one particular individual successfully making a case for sufficient resources to avoid him/her having to enter residential care. Having won the argument, there was a tendency for the individual then to be left to get on with it, with little help from their SSD. While the individuals interviewed who received direct or indirect payments were clearly doing a very good job of managing the purchase of personal assistance, they had received little assistance in making judgements about what were the most cost-effective and beneficial ways of using the money they had.

Such a situation may change with the full implementation of a care management system but SSDs will need to avoid what seems to be a common polarisation between either treating a disabled person as completely incapable of making their own decisions or assuming that they need no help at all in organising the purchase of personal assistance.

Breaking down barriers to independent living

Having control over the resources to pay for personal assistance is a necessary factor in creating opportunities for independent living but it is not sufficient. Those people in this study who were able to maximise the opportunities created were those who were also able to seek the advice and support of other disabled people who had similar experiences.

Being an employer is not easy, particularly for those people whose disabling experience leaves them with low self-esteem and provides little opportunity for developing the kind of skills necessary to be a good employer. The *Personal Assistance Users' Newsletter*, published by Hampshire Centre for Independent Living offers advice on the practicalities of being an employer, emphasising 'it is essential to be able to call on friends, perhaps a peer group, who can give you the support, advice and encouragement that you so desperately need ...' (*Personal Assistance Users' Newsletter*, September 1991, p. 7)

The disability movement, in publishing such newsletters, building up networks of support and, for example, running the Personal Assistance seminars put on by BCODP in 1992, is helping to create the confidence and skills amongst individual disabled people which will enable them to take full advantage of the opportunities offered by direct payments systems. Any social services authority which is serious about furthering the human and civil rights of disabled people will need to consider how to make such support possible for the personal assistance users (potential and current) in their own area.

Does independent living have a future?

It is clear from this study that having the money to pay for personal assistance is the most important factor in enabling disabled people to assert the kind of choices which non-disabled people take for granted. Those who were able to employ personal assistants had benefited from the establishment of the Independent Living Fund in 1988 and/or from the willingness of some local authority social services departments to make direct or indirect payments. Yet neither of these forms of direct payments systems has any future in the context of the community care reforms brought in by the 1990 legislation. It is to be hoped that some SSDs will continue to respond sympathetically to individuals' requests for direct/indirect payments, a small number will quality for grants from the new Fund which replaces the ILF and, of course, the 22 000 people who were in receipt of ILF grants in March 1993 will continue to receive funding from the ILF. Nevertheless, the focus of the community care reforms is on assessment by professionals as to what disabled people 'and their carers' need, purchase by care managers of the services deemed required, and delivery of services by health and social services statutory bodies or by private and voluntary sector organisations.

Although the stated philosophy of the government's approach to the community care reforms is 'helping people to live ... full and independent lives', the financial systems on which they are based actually take away choice. These financial systems are intended to take away the 'perverse incentive' for older and disabled people to enter residential care which had been created by entitlements under the social security system. The problem was created because the costs of residential care triggered the payment of social security benefits but the costs of assistance given at home did not. One option would have been to extend social security entitlements to cover the costs of personal assistance wherever it was given, a level playing field of the kind envisaged by the Wagner Committee:

> We have been much attracted by the idea of issuing Community Care Allowances to people with special needs, to be used by them to procure care servies of their choice. The allowance could be used either to recruit help in the home or to enter a residential home or – if preferred – could be banked with the area social services office where a nominated social worker could assemble a package of care services.

The Griffiths Report, and subsequently the government, rejected this option on the grounds that people's needs for assistance varied greatly:

> Our social security system is designed to provide a standard range of benefits for large numbers of people against objective tests of entitlement. It is not an appropriate system for the direct provision of individually tailored packages of support within a finite community care programme.

The Independent Living Fund of course showed that it was possible to operate a system where standard eligibility criteria triggered the right to a benefit but the level of payment was varied according to individual circumstance. The increase in demand on its budget, however, illustrated the most important barrier to incorporating such as system into the community care reforms – namely the cost implications for what Sir Roy Griffiths called 'a finite community care programme'.

There is no room for a fund such as the ILF, or for direct payments from SSDs, in the way that the community care reforms are being implemented. By closing the Fund to new applicants and insisting that potential applicants will instead have their personal assistance needs met by local authority services (with only a ,small number with very significant needs being able to receive a 'top up' grant from a new Fund) the government has reaffirmed the dominance of professional choice over the ability of disabled people to choose how their needs should be met. Both the Department of Health and the Treasury have continued to resist pressure to allow SSDs to make direct payments to individuals, insisting that social services authorities are concerned with delivering services and it is only the social security system which is concerned with making payments to individuals.

We have seen how disabled and older people are constructed as dependent people and how this has undermined their human and civil rights. In the context of the community care reforms, another socially constructed identity is being imposed on disabled and older people. They are now being seen as service users, with much emphasis on user involvement in the planning of services. While the rhetoric is about empowering people, it is difficult to be confident that this will happen when the one mechanism – direct payment systems – which clearly brings this about has no place in the reforms.

10

Prospects for the future

The research, policies and services which are concerned with the assistance that some people need to go about their daily lives have all used and abused the term 'care' in a way which is oppressive to those identified as being in need of 'care', those identified as 'dependent people'. Consequently, people who need physical assistance are being denied both human and civil rights.

Nevertheless, all is not doom and gloom. Even within the constraints imposed by the current shortage of resources, those responsible for implementing community care policies can act in ways which will make a major difference to disabled people's lives. The following points concern the kinds of changes which need to occur at the level of practitioners, statutory authorities and government in order to ensure that community care policies promote the human and civil rights of disabled people. It is important to realise that there is significant support for many of these changes, as is reflected in the advisory documents issued by the Department of Health's Community Care Support Force in March 1993 (see Community Care Support Force, 1993).

Changing attitudes

An important starting-point is to question the use of the terms 'carers', 'caring' and 'dependent people'. Those who need help with daily living activities cannot be treated with respect, their autonomy cannot be promoted, if their physical requirements are assumed to turn them into 'dependent people'. Neither can their personal relationships be respected if their partner, parent or relative is treated as a 'carer'.

We need to reclaim the words 'care' and 'caring' to mean 'love', to mean 'caring *about*' someone rather than 'caring *for*', with its custodial overtones.

When someone receives physical assistance from a paid worker or from a partner or relative, it is too often assumed that the 'caring' tasks carried out include taking responsibility for the person needing help. Rather than starting from this position – which is essentially a custodial one, a limiting of autonomy – service providers need to think about how disabled people's control over their lives can be promoted. It is not physical impairment which is the barrier to asserting choice and control. Rather, it is the obstacles which society constructs: the over-protectiveness of professionals and parents; the denial of education and employment opportunities; the undermining of self-esteem; the failure of non-disabled people to develop appropriate communication skills.

Service-led to needs-led assessments

A shift to assessment based on people's needs, rather than that determined by the type of services available, is seen as having a key role to play in achieving the White Paper's aim of helping people to lead 'full and independent lives'.

Disabled people have the right to ask for a comprehensive assessment of their needs (under the 1986 Disabled Persons Act) and social services authorities have a duty to meet any assessed needs for services which fall under Section 2 of the 1970 Chronically Sick and Disabled Persons Act. Financial constraints do not effect the statutory obligation to meet these needs.

However, social workers have, in the past, been directly and indirectly pressurised into limiting their assessments according to what can be provided in order to avoid legal action. If this is not to continue, and if assessments are to be genuinely needs-led rather than resource-led, then it is vital that assessment is carried out independently and separately from the allocation of resources. The rights of disabled people under the 1970 CSDP Act will only be furthered if assessors develop a professional ethic which is strong enough to resist pressure to assess according to the level of resources, and the type of services, available.

Self-assessment and advocacy services could have a key role to play in resisting the financial and organisational pressures to resource-led assessments. If disabled people are enabled to assess and articulate what they need to achieve a good quality of life, and if the assessment process becomes an effective channel of communication about need – unadulterated by professional assumptions about what need is and how it should be met – then community care policies are much more likely to promote human and civil rights.

The role of care management

Department of Health Policy Guidance states that 'it may be possible for some services users to play a more active part in their own care management, for example assuming responsibility for the day to day management of their carers may help to meet the aspirations of severely physically disabled people to be as independent as possible' (Department of Health, 1990, p.25). This possibility has been frequently offered to those disability organisations arguing for the legalisation of direct payments, as an alternative way of achieving choice and control over daily living.

The independent living movement is sceptical about the ability of a care management system to deliver the advantages of direct payment systems. However, if the government is serious about this alternative then it needs to more than merely remind social services departments of this possibility in its policy guidance. Disabled people should have the right to manage their own personal assistance requirements and should be given access to the wealth of expertise and experience which exists amongst those disabled people already involved in the daily practice of independent living.

The role of organisations of disabled people in service development and delivery

The government, health authorities and SSDs should be seeking out, and encouraging the development of, organisations controlled by disabled people. In the absence of purchasing power, such organisations are vital to the development of services which are determined by what people actually want. They have two particular contributions to make:

● influencing public and independent sector organisations to deliver services in a way which gives choice and control to the consumer of their services. The voice of disabled people needs to be much stronger at the level of planning services and, most importantly, at the level of contracting and contract-monitoring. Statutory authorities should not rely, as they have too often in the past, on isolated individuals to represent disabled people, but should seek out and encourage representative organisations of disabled people which, properly resourced, can make a valuable contribution.

creating a climate conducive to the growth of user-controlled service organisations. There are a few examples of organisations of disabled people which have successfully provided services which promote independent living. Such services usually originate as pilot projects. Three examples relevant to the current research are the Independent Living Advocate post at the National Spinal Injuries Centre, initiated by the Spinal Injuries Association and funded for two years by the Joseph Rowntree Foundation (see Morris, 1992b); the Haringey On-call Support Scheme, also initiated by the Spinal Injuries Association and funded by the King's Fund (see Zarb, forthcoming); and the Personal Assistance Advisor post initiated by Greenwich Association of Disabled People and funded by City Parochial and the Kings Fund, then by the joint finance mechanism (see Oliver and Zarb, 1992).

These projects have successfully demonstrated ways in which services controlled by disabled people create opportunities for independent living. Their survival, however, depends on the willingness of statutory authorities to purchase the service under the new contracting arrangements.

Both central government and health and social services authorities can help to bring about the major shift envisaged from service-led to needs-led provision by putting resources into organisations of disabled people to enable the voice of service users to be heard at all stages of community care implementation.

Direct payments

While the government has reminded SSDs that they should not be making payments to individuals, it is still possible to either set up a trust for this purpose (Eversley and Walsh, 1992) or to use voluntary organisations to administer grants for personal assistance. There is therefore room for SSDs to develop policies which incorporate the principles of independent living rather than the ideology of caring – and there is obviously considerable support for direct payments as the Association of Directors of Social Services passed a motion unanimously in favour of this in 1992. Moreover, there is increasing evidence that giving disabled people the cash to pay for personal assistance not only creates a better quality of life but is also a more cost effective way of meeting personal assistance needs than services provided by statutory organisations. Evaluation of the Personal Assistance Advisor post at Greenwich Association of Disabled People (GAD) found that, even when allowing for the cost of the support and advice given by the Personal Assistance Advisor, employing personal assistants was cheaper than relying on health and social services. Indeed this was a point recognised by Conservative Minister Nicholas Scott in his Foreword to the report when he wrote:

This report on Personal Assistance Schemes in Greenwich shows that as well as being cost effective, such schemes offer disabled people a greater degree of independence when compared with traditional forms of provision. (Oliver and Zarb, 1992)

A key feature of GAD's project is the provision of advocacy, advice and assistance to individuals employing their own personal assistants. It is clear that those people interviewed for this current research project who did not have access to the experience of other disabled people were not always getting value for their money. In particular, a reliance on agency staff – which is most common when the personal assistance user is soley dependent on social services professionals for advice – can mean paying a relatively large sum of money for a service which is quite restricted.

Having control over the resources to pay for personal assistance, therefore, is a necessary factor in creating opportunities for independent living but it is not sufficient. Those people in this study who were able to maximise the opportunities created were those who were able to seek the advice and support of other disabled people who had similar experiences.

Being an employer is not easy, particularly for people whose disabling experience leaves them with low self-esteem and provides little opportunity for developing the kind of skills necessary to be a good employer. The *Personal Assistance Users' Newsletter*, published by Hampshire Centre for Independent Living offers advice on the practicalities of being an employer, emphasising 'it is essential to be able to call on friends, perhaps a peer group, who can give you the support, advice and encouragement that you so desperately need' (*Personal Assistance Users' Newsletter*, September 1991, p.7).

The disability movement, in publishing such newsletters, building up networks of support, establishing Centres for Independent Living and, for example, running the Personal Assistance seminars put on by BCODP in 1992, is helping to create the confidence and skills amongst individual disabled people which will enable them to tackle the barriers to taking full advantage of the opportunities offered by direct payments systems. Any social services authority which is serious about furthering the human and civil rights of disabled people will need to consider how to make such support possible for the personal assistance users (potential and current) in their own area.

Questioning the current use of resources

It would appear that a shortage of resources is a major straitjacket on the extent to which community care reforms will promote independent living. However, it could be questioned as to whether the actual *level* of resources is the major problem or whether it is the nature of current service provision which ties up resources in particular ways which are incompatible with independent living. Changes driven by independent living principles could have major implications for the type of employment in the public and private sector and for provision which involves capital resources (Young Disabled Units, day centres, etc.) but it is not certain that the redistribution of resources which would be necessary would also need to be accompanied by an increase in the total amount of resources. Instead it may be that a fundamental shift in the use of existing resources would go a long way to acheiving independent living for disabled people.

Even in the case of the reliance on unpaid assistance provided by family members, which is said to save the government between £15bn and £24bn per year, it may be that once the wider, and indirect, costs of relying on family members are taken into account (lost tax revenues and national insurance contributions, greater expenditure on income support and other benefits, invalid care allowance, loss of productivity, etc.) that this is not in fact the cheap option it appears.

Conclusion

Over the last hundred years it has gradually become unacceptable to incarcerate disabled people in large institutions. The ideology of caring which is at the heart of current community care policies can only result in institutionalisation within the community unless politicians and professionals understand and identify with the philosophy and the aims of the independent living movement. Independent living is a human and civil rights issue; community care confines people to the four walls of their own home, preventing them from fully participating in personal relationships and in society, condoning the emotional and physical abuse which goes on behind closed doors.

While impairment is seen as necessarily creating dependency, as being a problem, a welfare issue for society to deal with, policies will always be at variance with disabled people's civil rights. Impairment and old age need to be seen as part of our (i.e. the whole society's) common experience. As an Australian Aboriginal woman once said 'If you have come to help me, then you can go back home. But if you see my struggle as part of your own survival then perhaps we can work together' (*Coalition*, September 1992, p.5).

Bibliography

Audit Commission (1986), *Making a Reality of Community Care* (London: HMSO)

Audit Commission (1987) *Community Care: Developing Services for People with a Mental Handicap* (London: HMSO).

Audit Commission (1992) *The Community Revolution: Personal Social Services and Community Care* (London: HMSO).

Baldwin, S. and Twigg, J. (1991) 'Women and community care: reflections on a debate' in M. McClean and D. Groves (eds) *Women's Issues in Social Policy* (London: Routledge).

Barnes, C. (1991) *Disabled People in Britain and Discrimination: A case for anti-discrimination legislation* (London: Hurst).

Barnes, M. and Wistow, G. (1991) *Changing Relationships in Community Care* (Leeds: Nuffield Institute for Health Service Studies).

Bayley, M. (1973) *Mental Handicap and Community Care* (London: Routledge & Kegan Paul).

Beardshaw, V. (1988) *Last on the List: Community Services for people with physical disabilities* (London: King's Fund Institute).

Beardshaw, V. (1992) *Implementing Assessment and Care Management: Learning from local experience 1990–1991* (London: King's Fund Institute).

Begum, N. (1990) *The Burden of Gratitude: Women with disabilities receiving personal care* (Warwick: University of Warwick and SCA).

Borsay, A. (1986) *Disabled People in the Community: A study of housing, health and welfare services* (London: Bedford Square Press).

Brechin, A. and Liddard, P. (eds) *Look at it this way* (Milton Keynes: Open University Press).

Brisenden, S. (1989) 'A charter for personal care' in *Progress*, 16 (Disablement Income Group).

Coalition, Quarterly journal produced by Greater Manchester Coalition of Disabled People.

Community Care Support Force (1993) *User Participation in Community Care Services*, A series of documents prepared by Jenny Morris and Vivien Lindow on behalf of the Community Care Support Force (Department of Health).

Conference of Socialist Economists State Group (1979) *Struggles over the State: Cuts and restructuring in contemporary Britain* (London: Conference of Socialist Economists Books).

Davis, K. (1981) 'Grove Road', *Disability Challenge* (Union of Physically Impaired Against Segregation).

Davis, K. (1988) 'Issues in Disability: Integrated Living' in *Social Problems and Social Welfare*, Workbook for Course D211, Block 3, Unit 19 (Milton Keynes: Open University Press).

Department of Health and Social Security (1981) *Growing Older* (London: HMSO).

Department of Health (1990) *Community Care in the Next Decade and Beyond: Policy guidance* (London: HMSO).

Department of Health (1991) *Getting it Right for Carers* (London: HMSO).

Equal Opportunities Commission (1982) *Who Cares for the Carers? Opportunities for those caring for the elderly and handicapped* (Manchester: EOC).

Eversley, J. and Walsh, B. (1992) Seminar on Independent Living Schemes: 24 June 1992 (unpublished background paper).

Fennell, G. Phillipson, C. and Evers, H. (eds) 1988 *The Sociology of Old Age* (Milton Keynes: Open University).

Fiedler, B. (1988) *Living Options Lottery: Housing and care support services for people with severe physical disability* (London: Prince of Wales Advisory Group on Disability).

Finch, J. (1984) 'Community Care: Developing Non-Sexist Alternatives' in *Critical Social Policy*, 9.

Finch, J. (1990) 'The Politics of Community Care in Britain' in C. Ungerson (ed.) *Gender and Caring: Work and Welfare in Britain and Scandinavia* (Hemel Hempstead: Harvester Wheatsheaf).

Finch, J. and Groves, D. (1983) *A Labour of Love: Women, Work and Caring* (London: Routledge & Kegan Paul).

Finkelstein, V. (1980) *Attitudes and Disabled People: Issues for Discussion* (New York: World Rehabilitation Fund).

Finkelstein, V. (1991) 'Disability: An administrative challenge? (The health and welfare heritage)', in M. Oliver (ed.) *Social Work: Disabled People and Disabling Environments* (London: Jessica Kingsley).

Glendinning, C. (1988) 'Dependency and Interdependency: The Incomes of Informal Carers and the Impact of Social Security' in S. Baldwin, G. Parker and R. Walker (eds) (1988) *Social Security and Community Care* (Aldershot: Gower).

Glendinning, C. (1992) *The Costs of Informal Care* (London: HMSO).

Graham, H. (1983) 'Caring: A labour of love' in Finch and Groves (eds) *A Labour of Love: Women, Work and Caring* (London: Routledge & Kegan Paul).

Groves, D. (1979), Letter in *New Society*, 20 September 1979.

Hampshire Centre for Independent Living (1986) *One Step On: Consumer-directed housing and care for disabled people – the experience of three people* (Petersfield: HCIL Publications).

Harrison, J. (1987) *Severe Physical Disability: Responses to the challenge of care* (London: Cassell).

Hevey, D. (1992) *The Creatures Time Forgot: Photography and disability imagery* (London: Routledge).

Hicks, C. (1988) *Who Cares: Looking after people at home* (London: Virago).
Humphries, S. and Gordon, P. (1992) *Out of Sight: The Experience of Disability 1900–1950* (Plymouth: Northcote).
Hunt, A. (1968) *A Survey of Women's Employment* (London: HMSO).
Hunt, A. (1978) *The Elderly at Home* (London HMSO).
Hunt, P. (1981) 'Settling Accounts with the Parasite People: a critique of *A Life Apart*', *Disability Challenge*, 1 (Union of the Physically Impaired against Segregation).
Hunter, D. J. and Judge, K. (1988) *Griffiths and Community Care: Meeting the Challenge* (London: King's Fund Institute).
Jones, K. Brown, J. and Bradshaw, J. (1983) *Issues in Social Policy*, (London: Routledge & Kegan Paul).
Keith, L. (1992) 'Who Cares Wins? Women, caring and disability' in *Disability, Handicap and Society*, volume 7, no 2, pp. 167–75.
Ann Kestenbaum (1992) *Cash for Care: A report on the experience of Independent Living Fund clients* (Nottingham: Independent Living Fund)
Land, H. (1978) 'Who cares for the family?', *Journal of Social Policy*, vol. 7, no. 3, pp. 357–84.
Lewis, J. and Meredith, B. (1988) *Daughters Who Care: Daughters caring for mothers at home* (London: Routledge).
Ann Macfarlane (1990) 'The Right to Make Choices' *Community Care*, 1 November 1990.
Mason, P. (1992), 'The Representation of Disabled People: a Hampshire Centre for Independent Living Discussion Paper' in *Disability Handicap and Society*, vol. 7, No 1, pp. 79–84.
McGlone, F. (1992) *Disability and Dependency in Old Age* (London: Family Policy Studies Centre).
McIntosh, M. (1979) 'The welfare state and the needs of the dependent family', in S. Burman (ed.) *Fit Work for Women* (London: Croom Helm).
Miller, E. J. and Gwynne, G. V. (1972) *A Life Apart* (London: Tavistock Publications).
Moroney, R. (1976) *The Family and the State* (London: Longmans).
Morris, A. and Butler, A. (1972) *No Feet to Drag* (London: Sedgewick & Jackson).
Morris, J. (1991) *Pride against Prejudice: Transforming attitudes towards disability* (London: The Women's Press).
Morris, J. (1992a) *Disabled Lives: Many Voices, One Message* (BBC Continuing Education Department).
Morris, J. (1992b), Interim Evaluation of the Post of Independent Living Advocate at the National Spinal Injuries Centre (unpublished report submitted to the Spinal Injuries Association).
National Audit Office (1987) *Community Care Developments* (London: NAO).
National Institute for Social Work (1988) *Residential Care: A positive choice* (London: HMS0).
Office of Population Censuses and Surveys (1988) *The Financial Circumstances of Disabled Adults Living in Private Households* (London: HMSO).

Oliver, J. and Briggs, A. (1983) *Caring: Experiences of looking after disabled relatives* (London: Routledge & Kegan Paul).

Oliver, M. (1990) *The Politics of Disablement* (Basingstoke: Macmillan).

Oliver, M. (1993) 'Disability, Citizenship and Empowerment' in *Workbook 2 for Course K665 The Disabling Society* (Milton Keynes: Open University Press).

Oliver, M. and Barnes, C. (1991) 'Discrimination, Disability and Welfare: From Needs to Rights', in I. Bynoe, M. Oliver and C. Barnes (1991) *Equal Rights for Disabled People: The case for a new law* (London: IPPR).

Oliver, M. and Zarb, G. (1992) *Greenwich Personal Assistance Schemes: Second Year Evaluation* (London: Greenwich Association of Disabled People).

Oswin, M. (1992) 'The Carer's Tale' in *Community Care*, 16 July 1992, pp. 16–17.

Pagel, M. (1988) *On Our Own Behalf* (Manchester: GMCDP Publications).

Parker, G. (1992) *With this body: Caring and disability in marriage* (Buckingham: Open University Press).

Personal Assistance Users' Newsletter, monthly newsletter produced by Hampshire Centre for Independent Living (available from HCIL, 4 Plantation Way, Whitehill, Bordon, Hants, GU35 9HD).

Pitkeathley, J. (1989) *It's My Duty, Isn't It? The plight of carers in our society* (London: Souvenir Press).

Qureshi, H. and Walker, A. (1989) *The Caring Relationship: Elderly people and their families* (London: Macmillan).

RADAR and Arthritis Care (1991) *The Right to a Clean Home* (London: RADAR and Arthritis Care).

Ratzka, A. (1986) *Independent Living and Attendant Care in Sweden: A consumer perspective* (Monograph).

Royal College of Physicians (1986) *The Young Disabled Adult: The use of residential homes and hospital units for the age group 16–64* (London: Royal College of Physicians).

Social Services Inspectorate (1987) *From Home Help to Home Care: An Analysis of Policy, Resourcing and Service Management* (Department of Health).

Social Services Inspectorate (1991a), *Getting the Message Across: A guide to developing and communicating policies, principles and procedures on assessment* (London: HMSO).

Social Services Inspectorate (1991b) *Care Management and Assessment: Summary of Practice Guidance* (London: HMSO).

Towsend, P. (1986) 'Ageism and Social Policy' in Phillipson, C. and Walker, A. (eds) *Ageing and Social Policy* (Aldershot: Gower).

Twigg, J. Atkin, K. and Perring, C. (1990) *Carers and Services: A review of research* (London: HMSO).

Ungerson, C. (1987) *Policy is Personal: Sex, Gender and Informal Care* (London: Tavistock).

Ungerson, C. (ed.) (1990) *Gender and Caring: Work and welfare in Britain and Scandinavia* (Hemel Hempstead: Harvester Wheatsheaf).

Wilkinson, S. and Hughes, D. (1992) *Care Free? An Evaluation of the Independent Living Fund* (Bristol: United Bristol Healthcare Trust).
Wilson, E. (1977) *Women and the Welfare State* (London: Tavistock).
Wood, R. (1991) 'Caring for disabled people' in G. Dalley (ed.) *Disability and Social Policy* (London: Policy Studies Institute).
Working Group on Joint Planning (1985) *Progress in Partnership* (London: DHSS).
Zarb, G. (forthcoming, 1993) *Evaluation of Haringey On-Call Support Scheme* (King's Fund/Spinal Injuries Association).

Index